Dosages and Calculations

Dosages and Calculations

Second Edition

RICHARD WIEDERHOLD

JONES AND BARTLETT PUBLISHERS

Sudbury, Massachusetts

BOSTON   TORONTO   LONDON   SINGAPORE

World Headquarters
Jones and Bartlett Publishers
40 Tall Pine Drive
Sudbury, MA 01776
978-443-5000
info@jbpub.com
www.jbpub.com

Jones and Bartlett Publishers
Canada
6339 Ormindale Way
Mississauga, Ontario L5V 1J2
Canada

Jones and Bartlett Publishers
International
Barb House, Barb Mews
London W6 7PA
United Kingdom

Jones and Bartlett's books and products are available through most bookstores and online book-sellers. To contact Jones and Bartlett Publishers directly, call 800-832-0034, fax 978-443-8000, or visit our website www.jbpub.com.

Substantial discounts on bulk quantities of Jones and Bartlett's publications are available to corporations, professional associations, and other qualified organizations. For details and specific discount information, contact the special sales department at Jones and Bartlett via the above contact information or send an email to specialsales@jbpub.com.

The author, editor, and publisher have made every effort to provide accurate information. However, they are not responsible for errors, omissions, or for any outcomes related to the use of the contents of this book and take no responsibility for the use of the products and procedures described. Treatments and side effects described in this book may not be applicable to all people; likewise, some people may require a dose or experience a side effect that is not described herein. Drugs and medical devices are discussed that may have limited availability controlled by the Food and Drug Administration (FDA) for use only in a research study or clinical trial. Research, clinical practice, and government regulations often change the accepted standard in this field. When consideration is being given to use of any drug in the clinical setting, the health care provider or reader is responsible for determining FDA status of the drug, reading the package insert, and reviewing prescribing information for the most up-to-date recommendations on dose, precautions, and contraindications, and determining the appropriate usage for the product. This is especially important in the case of drugs that are new or seldom used.

Production Credits

Publisher: David Cella
Editorial Assistant: Maro Asadoorian
Production Manager: Julie Champagne Bolduc
Production Assistant: Jessica Steele Newfell
Associate Marketing Manager: Lisa Gordon
Manufacturing and Inventory Control
  Supervisor: Amy Bacus

Composition: International Typesetting and
  Composition
Cover Design: Anne Spencer
Assistant Photo Researcher: Meghan Hayes
Cover Image: © AbleStock
Printing and Binding: Malloy, Inc.
Cover Printing: Malloy, Inc.

Photo Credits
Figure 9-3 and Figure 9-4 Courtesy of Armstrong Medical Industries, Inc.

Library of Congress Cataloging-in-Publication Data
Wiederhold, Richard.
  Dosages and calculations/Richard Wiederhold. — 2nd ed.
    p. ; cm.
  Rev. ed. of: Brady dosages and calculations/Richard Wiederhold. c1992.
  Includes bibliographical references and index.
  ISBN 978-0-7637-4985-9 (pbk. : alk. paper)
  1. Pharmaceutical arithmetic. I. Wiederhold, Richard. Brady dosages and calculations. II. Title.
  [DNLM: 1. Pharmaceutical Preparations—administration & dosage—Programmed Instruction.
  2. Mathematics—Programmed Instruction. QV 18.2 W644d 2009]
  RS57.W54 2009
  615'.1401513—dc22
                          2008037526
6048

Printed in the United States of America
12 11 10 09 08   10 9 8 7 6 5 4 3 2 1

Contents

Foreword

For those of us who work in or around the edges of medical science, there is such a terrible temptation to feel quite satisfied with our progress. Every issue of the leading professional journals, for example, includes evidence of some advance in the techniques, the technologies, or the chemistry of medicine. Particularly in the constant evolution of chemical responses to disease do we get the impression that our society enjoys some kind of superior status.

In reality, an enormous body of information regarding medicine was acquired before medicine was ever recognized as a science. As this book points out, there are only five sources of medication: animal, vegetable, mineral, electrical, and synthetic.

Throughout the history of our species, remedies derived from animal, vegetable, and mineral sources have been applied to countless willing and unwilling subjects. Thousands of years before the creation of scientific journals—indeed, before the invention of paper—primitive folk healers were experimenting with substances and compounds that were readily available. Their outcomes were reported verbally and passed from generation to generation.

The author of this book acknowledges the contention that there may be thousands of undiscovered medically beneficial plants growing in the Amazon River basin alone. For the time being, however, most of our scientific attention is directed toward the creation and manufacture of synthetic drugs—resulting from either chemical reactions or gene-splicing techniques.

As this book was nearing the final stages of publication, we were reminded that scientific progress on the one hand can become meaningless in the face of erroneous or negligent human performance. A report in a major medical journal revealed that medication errors—including dosage calculations—were occurring in a frightfully large number of cases at one teaching hospital. The assumption was that the experience of that hospital and its patients was typical.

That report reminded me of a time nearly 20 years ago. I was the supervisor of some of America's first paramedic trainees, and I witnessed their difficult absorption of a whole new body of technical information, including pharmacology and dosage calculations. The books and reference materials they were expected to use were not student friendly, and I worried about their potential for immediate recall and accurate performance while working with critical patients in the inhospitable environment of street medicine.

The most advanced therapeutic compound is of no value unless it is administered accurately. The chemical valence of a revolutionary compound is irrelevant unless the people who administer that compound are sufficiently schooled and skilled to calculate the dosage.

This book promises to be a valuable tool for both the student and the practitioner. Written in straightforward, plain English, it avoids the unnecessary jargon and techno-babble that so often confound the reader. I only wish it had been available for my paramedic trainees 20 years ago.

While we tend to view the folk medicine of early human history as primitive, we are quick to overlook the fact that many of today's patients get lost or damaged in the assembly-line processes of "modern" medicine. With the kind of commonsense presentation of facts and procedures Rich Wiederhold offers in this book, we can bridge the gap between scientific advance and reliable human application.

James Page, JD

Acknowledgments

I wish to thank the fine folks at Jones and Bartlett without whom this project would not have been possible. Their help and guidance was instrumental in bringing you a quality product. Special thanks go to Dave Cella, who believed in the project and offered me a contract to publish; Maro Asadoorian, editorial assistant, who kept me on track; Jess Newfell, production assistant, who was a pleasant voice on the other end of the telephone; Michelle Cain, who tediously copyedited the text and made many improvements; and Scarlett Stoppa, who proofread the text. Their collective efforts were essential to this project, and I thank them all. Lastly I want to thank the late Jim Page for his eloquent preface to the book. Jim, your legacy in EMS will not be forgotten.

Chapter 1

Introduction to Dosage Calculations

> There is
> no such thing as a problem
> without a gift for you
> in its hands.
>
> You seek problems
> because you need
> their gifts.
>
> —Richard Bach. *Illusions: Confessions of a Reluctant Messiah*. New York:
>   Bantam Dell Publishing Group; 1977.

Exhibit 1-1

This text begins with simple mathematical problems and creates a bridge from the known to the unknown. Each chapter builds on information from previous chapters. Look ahead through the work. Do not be intimidated by the advanced problems. Master the objectives, taking one step at a time toward completion.

This text will prepare the reader to calculate correct doses of medications. Mathematical skills are necessary to master the material. These include simple skills of addition, subtraction, multiplication, and division. Slightly more complex skills include factoring and use of whole numbers, mixed numbers, decimal numbers, negative numbers, and fractions. They also include converting from one unit (such as hours) to another (such as minutes). The ability to solve simple ratio equations to determine one unknown factor is also necessary.

Many calculations in this text can be easily derived intuitively, in one's thoughts, without setting up an equation. There are problems with using this shortcut of intuitive deduction. The text will progressively build from simple and easily solved problems to more complex problems. Complex problems will require equations for their solution. Practice with the early, simple problems will prepare the clinician to set up and solve later, more complex ones. Solving problems intuitively is good practice. Go ahead and get an intuitive answer. Then set up an equation to solve for the same answer and check the calculations.

Most problems presented in this text represent doses of actual medications. They are usually American Heart Association–Advanced Cardiac Life Support medications and doses.

The text has attempted as much as possible to avoid gender-specific pronouns. However, whenever syntax made it necessary, the masculine pronouns *his* or *he* are used to simplify grammatical structure. This is a standard grammatical convention and in no way is intended to slight female patients, physicians, or clinicians.

That is the beginning of Knowledge,
the discovery of something
we do not understand.

—Frank Herbert. *Dune.* Randor, PA: Children Book Company; 1965.

Exhibit 1-2

OBJECTIVES

Upon completion of this chapter the clinician should be able to:

1. Discuss patient rights in receiving medication
2. Discuss patient rights to privacy as provided by the HIPAA Privacy Rule
3. Discuss the health care professional's responsibilities in administering medication
4. Identify regulating agencies and legislation regarding medication
5. Discuss origins and major classifications of medication
6. Identify how medication is supplied, including pills, tablets, capsules, prefilled syringes, ampules, vials, etc.
7. Discuss factors influencing dosage, such as patient weight, age, sex, allergies, medical history, pregnancy, and concomitant medications
8. Discuss untoward effects of medication, including dependence, side effects, tolerance, and idiosyncratic reactions
9. Differentiate between parenteral and nonparenteral routes of administration and related rates of adsorption into the body systems

10. Discuss the therapeutic envelope, including subtherapeutic doses and toxic doses

11. Discuss the risk of transmission of infectious diseases associated with administering medication and techniques with which the clinician may reduce risk

KEY TERMS

acquired tolerance
addiction
affect
allergy
ampule
anaphylactic reaction
antibiotic
antidepressant
antidysrhythmic
antihistamine
antihypertensive
antihypoglycemic
barbiturate
behavioral toxicity
cardiotonic
chemical name
chemotherapy
chronotropic
concomitant
confidentiality
dependence
depressant
diuretic
dose
effect
elixir
endotracheal instillation
ethics
FDA
first pass effect
generic name
habituation

hallucinogen
hypersensitivity
hypnotic
informed consent
inotropic
inscription
intracardiac
intradermal
intramuscular
intraosseous
intravenous
MedicAlert
medicine
mineral origin
mucosa
narcotic
nonparenteral
organic
overdose
parenteral
PDR
percutaneous
potentiation
rate
recombinant DNA therapy
serum
side effect
sign
signature
solution
stimulant
subcutaneous

sublingual	tolerance
subscription	toxic
superscription	trade name
suppository	tranquilizer
synergism	untoward effect
synthetic origin	vaccine
syringe	vasopressor
therapeutic	vial
therapeutic envelope	withdrawal

CASE STUDY

The fire department lieutenant received the call while he was on duty. There were no emergencies at the moment, so he called in a replacement to cover his position. The call was that his teenage daughter, who had been sick with a cold, had developed a fever, so his wife took her to the emergency department of the local hospital to be examined and medicated. There was no urgency or rush, but the lieutenant wanted to stop by and make sure his daughter was OK. It took about an hour for his replacement to arrive. As he left the office, the phone was ringing, but he didn't stop because he knew his replacement could handle whatever was coming in. He forgot his cell phone in his hurry to get to the hospital. He didn't speed. He arrived and entered the emergency department. People he knew and worked with every day were quiet. No one made eye contact with him. A chaplain met him and asked him to join him in the church chapel. This alerted him that something was seriously wrong. He asked, "Where's my wife? How is my daughter?" "She's in the chapel," the chaplain replied, "and your daughter is what we need to talk about." In the chapel his wife was crying quietly. Minutes later he learned his daughter was dead. The tragedy of her death stunned him and his wife. They couldn't understand why she had died from a cold. Was this some kind of rare virus? Did they miss something about her illness? Did they contribute to her death by not insisting she go to the doctor sooner? All the staff could tell them was that they gave her an antibiotic for her illness, and she seized and went into cardiac arrest with **signs** of **anaphylactic reaction**. Their words were guarded, and they would not say more than the very basics of what had happened. He asked what antibiotic they had given her. The answer chilled his heart. The hospital staff had given his daughter a medication to which she was acutely allergic. The joy of his life was now dead because somebody prescribed and somebody else gave a medication without reading the patient's chart or asking the sick but very alert teenager about her allergies. She would never graduate, never marry, never have children, and never come home again.

INTRODUCTION

This is a true case study with slight modifications! As you study this text, try to imagine how the clinician who gave that medication feels about the mistake, and remember your responsibilities when you calculate and give a dose.

Any text that proposes to deal with the topic of dosage calculations is obligated to address more than the mathematical calculations required to derive the correct **dose**. Many other issues—such as the patient's rights, the clinician's responsibilities, the **effects** of drugs, how the drugs work, and how they are administered—are included. The concept of rights and responsibilities is a primary one to the act of administering medications and serves here as the introduction to this book.

PATIENT RIGHTS

Every mentally competent adult living in a democratic society has the right to refuse or discontinue medical treatment at any time. This concept dates to one of the earliest human rights documents—the Magna Carta, signed by King John in 1215—which stated:

> No freeman shall be taken, or imprisoned, or outlawed, or exiled, or in any way harmed, nor will we go upon him nor will we send upon him, except by the legal judgment of his peers or by the law of the land.[1]

A patient receiving a medication must give **informed consent** to be treated before receiving the medication. Case law defining a patient's right to refuse treatment dates to 1767. Justice Cordorzo ruled in a case involving New York Hospital in 1914:

> Every human being of adult years and sound mind has a right to determine what should be done with his own body; and a surgeon who performs an operation without his patient's consent commits an assault for which he is liable in damages.[2]

The National Commission for the Protection of Human Subjects of Biomedical and Behavioral Research identified in its Belmont Report three

---

[1] Magna Carta (1215).
[2] New York Circuit Court Ruling (1914). Justice Cordorzo.

conditions for consent to be "informed." These include information, comprehension, and voluntariness as paraphrased here:

> The patient should be given accurate information, in simple language about the treatment, its potential risks and benefits, and alternatives. The patient must comprehend the information given. Informed consent may only be granted by a competent adult who understands the information provided. This condition may not be properly met if the information is presented in too technical a manner, a language in which the patient is not fluent, or to a patient who is emotionally or mentally impaired by alcohol, drug abuse, or health disabilities.[3]

Voluntariness means the consent must be made without coercion. There should be no excessive pressure or reward for the patient's consent.

Clinical human research has been recognized as an important method of obtaining information about disease and treatment. The rights of patients to be informed of and participate in an experiment must also be protected. The Nuremberg Code and the Declaration of Helsinki define conditions for human research. The National Commission for the Protection of Human Subjects of Biomedical and Behavioral Research reinforces this concept.

Patients also have a right to **confidentiality** (privacy) regarding their medical care. Health care providers may discuss a patient's medical information with other providers. In fact, they have a responsibility to do so. However, a patient's medical information should not be discussed with persons not involved in the patient's care. Clinicians should not discuss a patient where they may be overheard. This is a violation of the patient's right to confidentiality.

Some states define situations in which a patient does not have a right to confidentiality. These usually include gunshot wounds and child abuse. Child abuse is excepted from confidentiality on the basis that the victim is not a competent adult and can only be protected if the abuse is reported. Gunshot wounds are usually excepted because assault with a deadly weapon is a felony and requires being reported by law.

The U.S. Department of Health and Human Services issued the Privacy Rule to implement federal legislation passed in 1996. That legislation was the Health Insurance Portability and Accountability Act (HIPAA). HIPAA caused a stir in the health community workplace as providers took steps to

---

[3] Spivery, W. H. (1989, July). Informed consent for clinical research in the emergency department. *Annals of Emergency Medicine.* 18(7).

ensure the privacy of patient records and to inform patients of their privacy rights. (It is beyond the scope of this text to provide a legal definition of the act. The act can be accessed at http://www.hhs.gov/ocr/hipaa. The information presented here is a simplified overview and should not be used as a guideline for policy development.)

HIPAA identifies protected health information (PHI) that agencies governed by the act must keep confidential for patients. Those agencies are called "covered entities." Covered entities may include hospitals, emergency medical service providers, physical therapy centers, medical insurance plans (including private, government, and charitable plans), and others. PHI includes any individually identifiable health information held or transmitted by a covered entity or its business associate, in any form or media, whether electronic, paper, or oral.

Most employing agencies that are covered entities now have organizational policies in place to ensure that employees comply with HIPAA. A clinician who has questions should refer to both the act and his employer, to understand the employer's interpretation of the act. Nothing in the act prohibits disclosing information to the individual patient.

HIPAA permits disclosure of protected information to law enforcement under six circumstances:

> Covered entities may disclose protected health information to law enforcement officials for law enforcement purposes under the following six circumstances, and subject to specified conditions: (1) as required by law (including court orders, court-ordered warrants, subpoenas) and administrative requests; (2) to identify or locate a suspect, fugitive, material witness, or missing person; (3) in response to a law enforcement official's request for information about a victim or suspected victim of a crime; (4) to alert law enforcement of a person's death, if the covered entity suspects that criminal activity caused the death; (5) when a covered entity believes that protected health information is evidence of a crime that occurred on its premises; and (6) by a covered health care provider in a medical emergency not occurring on its premises, when necessary to inform law enforcement about the commission and nature of a crime, the location of the crime or crime victims, and the perpetrator of the crime.[4]

---

[4] U.S. Department of Health and Human Services, Office of Civil Rights. *HIPPAHIPAA: Medical Privacy National Standards to Protect the Privacy of Personal Health Information*. Retrieved July 24, 2008, from http://www.hhs.gov/ocr/privacysummary.pdf.

HIPAA provides a criminal penalty: "A person who knowingly obtains or discloses individually identifiable health information in violation of HIPAA faces a fine of $50,000 and up to one-year imprisonment."[5]

Violating a patient's rights is not usually a criminal act. A violation of criminal law is either a misdemeanor or a felony. Violation of a person's rights is a tort. To remedy a tort, restitution is sought in a civil court, rather than with police officers and a criminal court.

Medical ethics are an important consideration for any clinician who gives medication. **Ethics** is the study of right and wrong. There are no clearly defined absolutes of what a clinician should do. Ethical decisions about health care may be guided by civil law but usually result from individual decisions. General Robert E. Lee summed it up when he said, "Do your duty in all things. You cannot do more, you should never wish to do less."[6]

One guide to medical ethics is the Oath of Geneva (Exhibit 1-3), developed by the World Health Organization in 1948.

I solemnly pledge myself to consecrate my life to the service of humanity; I will give to my teachers the respect and gratitude which is their due; I will practice my profession with consciency and dignity; the health of my patient will be my first consideration; I will respect the secrets which are confided in me; I will maintain by all the means in my power the honor and noble traditions of the medical profession; my colleagues will be my brothers; I will not permit considerations of religion, nationality, race, party politics, or social standing to intervene between my duty and my patient; I will maintain the utmost respect for human life from the time of conception; even under threat, I will not make use of my medical knowledge contrary to the laws of humanity. I make these promises solemnly, freely, and upon my honor.

—Adopted by the General Assembly of the World Medical Association, Geneva, Switzerland (1948, September). Amended by the 22nd World Medical Assembly, Sydney, Australia (1968, August).

Exhibit 1-3 Oath of Geneva

THE CLINICIAN'S RESPONSIBILITIES

All medication doses should be recorded in the patient's chart or report. This chart or report is a legal document and medication administration record. Legal documents are admissible as evidence in a court of law.

---

[5] Ibid.

[6] Custis Lee, G. W. (1852, April 5). Letter to his son. Published in *The New York Sun* on November 26, 1864. Also inscribed beneath his bust in the Hall of Fame on the former New York University campus in New York City.

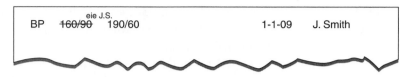

Figure 1-1 Sample Chart

There are standard accepted practices in medical charting. Violation of these practices will work to the charting clinician's disadvantage in a malpractice legal action. The clinician will have to explain why the chart was not completed properly. An opposing attorney may imply there are only two valid reasons: incompetence or dishonesty.

Charting practices are based on common sense and are intended to standardize charts' contents. Nothing should be erased, whited out, obscured, or added at a later date to change a chart unless the change is clearly documented.

When changes are required, the clinician should mark through any error with a single line. He should not completely obscure the error. The correction should then be made. The chart should also be marked with the notation EIE (for "entered in error") (Figure 1-1) or the indication "error" and the initials of the person making the correction. It is not acceptable to write over an error, thereby correcting it, such as in changing a 7 to a 9. Writing over an entry may raise doubts about which number was correct and why a correction was not made in the standard way. Additions should be made in the same manner and should include a date indicating the notation is an addition.

Medications given in a dose that is less than a whole number should be recorded with a zero before the decimal to avoid error.

For example: A patient receives two pills of 0.5 g of medication in each pill. The chart would read "gave 1 g in two pills of 0.5 g each" of whatever medication is administered.

The written record of medication given to a patient should always be initialed by the person giving the medication. The first initial and the last name is the most appropriate chart entry in this case. The time, date, and reaction (or absence of one) to the **medicine** should also be recorded whenever possible.

REGULATION AND STANDARDIZATION OF MEDICINE

The federal Food and Drug Administration, known as the **FDA**, is a division of the U.S. Department of Health and Human Services. The FDA was established by the federal Food, Drug, and Cosmetic Act of 1938 and subsequent, related legislation.

The FDA periodically visits, inspects, and collects samples from drug-manufacturing and storage facilities. The samples then are analyzed at one of the FDA's 19 district laboratories for quality, purity, and correct labeling.

The FDA must approve any new products offered for sale or interstate traffic in the United States. New medications and medications from other countries must meet a thorough approval process before being marketed in the United States.

The Harrison Narcotic Act of 1914 set up regulation for narcotics and other controlled substances. It was amended, to increase the list of controlled substances and to increase penalties for illegal trafficking, in 1956 by the Narcotic Control Act.

The Bureau of Narcotics and Dangerous Drugs was an agency of the Department of Justice that kept a registry of physicians who were permitted to give out or prescribe controlled substances. It was replaced by the Drug Enforcement Agency (DEA) in the Controlled Substances Act of 1970. The DEA issues a registration number to each physician who is licensed to dispense controlled medications.

Parts of a Prescription

A prescription is an order written by a physician, dentist, or practitioner licensed to prescribe medication. It authorizes a pharmacist to dispense medications regulated and controlled by the FDA under the federal Food, Drug, and Cosmetic Act.

A prescription has four format components: the inscription, the subscription, the superscription, and the signature.

- The **inscription** is the body of the prescription. It contains the name of the medication, its concentration, the form of the drug (pill, liquid, etc.), and the dose.
- The **subscription** is directions to the pharmacist about preparation of the medication.
- The **superscription** is the "Rx" symbol. It literally translates as "take thou."
- The **signature** includes the physician's signature and instructions to the patient. It also includes general information, such as the physician's address and narcotic registry number, the date, and whether the prescription may be refilled.

Standards of Medications

The *Physician's Desk Reference*, also know as the **PDR**, is an unofficial reference text published annually. It is a compilation of information concerning drugs, including indications, dosages, precautions, **side effects**, contraindications, etc. The information is essentially the same as that included in the package insert required by the FDA in prescription medications.

The standards for drugs are published in the *United States Pharmacopeia* (USP) every five years. It has included the National Formulary since 1975. The USP is the authorized source of information on drugs, their chemical composition, quality tests, storage requirements, and their preparation. The USP is prepared under supervision of a national committee of pharmacists, pharmacologists, physicians, chemists, biologists, and other scientific and allied personnel. The *United States Pharmacopeia* was adopted as standard in 1906.

ORIGINS OF MEDICATIONS

There are five origins of medication: animal, vegetable, mineral, synthetic, and electrical. Electrical energy is more correctly a therapy rather than a medication. It is addressed here because electrical therapies have doses of energy that must be calculated.

Animal origin includes all medicines, serums, and vaccines developed from human or animal origin. Insulin is an example of a medication once made only from pig and cow pancreases. It is now synthetically produced. Most medications of animal origin are either vaccines or serums.

Vaccines are **solutions** containing infectious agents. The intent is to administer an infectious agent to the patient to stimulate the patient's own immune system to generate antibodies to combat future infections. The infectious agents used as vaccines are deliberately weakened before injection to avoid giving the patient the disease. Vaccines are used prophylactically to prevent infection.

Serums are made by vaccinating lab animals, such as horses or human volunteers, with less-than-fatal doses of a disease organism. This allows the animal to create antibodies. Blood with the desired antibodies is then removed from the animal, processed, and used as a serum to treat others who have contracted or been exposed to the disease. Antivenin for the treatment of snakebites is an example of a serum.

Vegetable origin includes all medications derived from plants and plant products. For many years it was known that a tea made from the foxglove plant helped patients with chest pain. Modern research discovered the active ingredient of the foxglove was digitalis. Digitalis is now one of the most prescribed medications for cardiac patients.

Many other medications have been derived from plant products. Penicillin was discovered as a mold growing on bread. Aspirin, opium, quinine, reserpine, and ergot are other plant products.

The Amazon River basin has contributed many medications. Many environmentalists believe there may be thousands of undiscovered medically beneficial plants in the Amazon River basin alone.

Mineral origin includes necessary vitamins and minerals, such as calcium, iron, and potassium. Boric acid, Epsom salts, and iodine are other medications of mineral origin.

Synthetic origin drugs are manufactured in a laboratory. These include medications created by chemical reactions or by gene-splicing techniques.

Recombinant DNA therapy origin is the name given to gene-splicing techniques that create new organisms. Scientists have been able to introduce genes into some bacteria or yeast to make them produce something new. Human insulin is now being created by recombinant DNA therapy. Eli Lilly and Company has the trademark Humulin, which is an insulin product "structurally identical to the insulin produced by your body's pancreas."[7]

The advantage to this is that a more pure product with fewer side effects can be manufactured. There is a lower incidence of allergic sensitivity. As a synthesized product, it can be produced in a non-disease-producing laboratory without the risk of using blood serums that have undetected bloodborne disease.

Recombivax is a trademark medication of Merck & Co. It is a vaccine of recombinant DNA therapy against hepatitis B. Older forms of the anti-hepatitis B vaccine were made from the blood serum of professional blood donors, whose profit motive may have encouraged inaccurate reporting of health risk factors. With the advent of human immunodeficiency virus (HIV) and its associated disease, acquired immunodeficiency syndrome (AIDS), health care providers were concerned about the possibility of undetected disease in the blood serums. The development of synthetic medication eliminates the possibility of an undetected infection being present in donor blood.

As mentioned earlier, electrical origin is not actually a medication. It is more correctly a therapy. Electrical energy is measured in doses and may interact

---

[7] Eli Lilly and Company. *Information for the Patient: Humulin N (NPH Human Insulin).* Retrieved July 24, 2008, from http://pi.lilly.com/us/humulin-n-ppi.pdf.

with other medications, especially digitalis, so it will be addressed in this text. Electrical energy is used to control abnormal heart rhythms (dysrhythmias) by shocking the heart to regulate its rate or to convert the rhythm to a more normal one.

CLASSIFICATIONS OF MEDICATION

Medications are commonly classified in many ways. Two of the most common are by their actions or by their composition.

In the United States, medications are either controlled and available only by prescription or less stringently controlled and available over-the-counter without a prescription. Any medication or drug may be abused. Abuse is use of a medicine in a manner other than required for therapeutic management of an illness or injury.

Antibiotics are medications used to counter infections by bacterial microorganisms.

Antidepressants are used to counter emotional depression. These usually produce central nervous system depression.

Antidysrhythmics regulate or improve heart rhythm. These may be prescribed prophylactically, to prevent abnormal rhythms, or reactively, to treat existing abnormal rhythms.

Antihistamines counter histamine actions. These are used by persons suffering from some gastric ailments, allergies, and hay fever. Many antihistamines are sold over-the-counter.

Antihypertensives are a group of medications that counter high blood pressure (hypertension).

Antihypoglycemics are medications that stimulate insulin secretion in patients with Type II diabetes.

Barbiturates are **organic** compounds derived from barbituric acid. These are central nervous system **depressants** and highly addictive. They are used to induce sleep, relieve pain, and control seizure activity.

Cardiotonics are medications that improve the contractility (or rate) of the heart.

Chronotropics are medications that affect the heart rate.

Diuretics are medications that stimulate the production of urine. These are used in patients with diseases, such as congestive heart failure, that result in too much fluid in the body.

Hallucinogens induce hallucinations. Hallucinations are false sensory perceptions, such as seeing visions, hearing voices, feeling something, etc. Hallucinogens are frequently abused for recreational use. Lysergic acid diethylamide (LSD) was a popular hallucinogen in the 1960s. It is still an abused drug but is less popular now.

Hypnotics are sedatives that induce sleep. Some hypnotics are also barbiturates. *Hypnotic* refers to the medication's actions, while *barbiturate* refers to its composition.

Inotropic medications are cardiotonics that increase the contractility of the heart.

Narcotics depress the central nervous system. They relieve pain, induce sleep, and in excessive doses, produce coma and death. Narcotics are addictive, controlled medications. Heroin is an addictive narcotic derived from morphine. Its importation, sale, and use in the United States are illegal. Medical scientists agree its pharmacokinetic actions can be accomplished by other, less addictive drugs.

Stimulants are medications that increase the target organ's activity. Amphetamines are central nervous system stimulants that are sometimes prescribed as diet pills. They are commonly abused and illegally purchased from uncontrolled sources. Cocaine is another highly popular, dangerous, addictive stimulant of abuse.

Tranquilizers reduce anxiety and mental tension. This may have the indirect effect of enabling the anxious patient to sleep. Tranquilizers are psychologically and physically addicting. They are frequently unintentionally abused. It is difficult to achieve the appropriate level of relaxation without side effects of drowsiness, slowed reactions, and occasionally emotional depression.

Vasopressors are medications that cause the contraction of the capillaries and raise resistance to the flow of blood. This causes an increase in blood pressure.

Other major categories of medications include analgesic, anesthetic, antiepileptic, antifungal, antipyretic, antispasmodic, antitussive, bronchodilator, cathartic, cholinergic, and many more.

HOW MEDICATION IS IDENTIFIED

Every legal medication in the United States is labeled. The medication label provides important information, including trade name, generic name, strength or concentration, number or amount of medication units, expiration date, usual dosage, special precautions, and manufacturer's name.

The **trade name** is given to a medication by its manufacturer. This is marked by a small *R* enclosed by a circle (®). This symbol means the name is a registered trademark. The first letter of a trade name is capitalized. Different pharmaceutical companies may give different trade names to the same medication.

The **generic name** is given to the medication by the first manufacturer or discoverer. It is usually related to the drug's chemical structure. (This text will use the generic name for medications.) The **chemical name** reflects the drug's chemical structure. This name is derived with firmly established scientific guidelines. It reflects the exact chemical makeup of the medication.

The *United States Pharmacopeia* is the authorized treatise on drugs in the United States.

Exhibit 1-4 *United States Pharmacopeia*

HOW MEDICATIONS ARE SUPPLIED

Oral medications may be supplied as round tablets (such as aspirin), elongated tablets, or capsules. Occasionally, a tablet is coated to facilitate its adsorption or cause a time-released effect. Capsules are cylindrical-shaped gelatin containers that enclose a single dose of medication, sometimes a liquid or suspension. The purpose of the capsule is to protect the patient from an unpleasant taste while taking the medicine.

Injectable medications may be supplied as prefilled single-dose **syringes**, **ampules**, or multiple dose **vials**. Prefilled syringes have the advantage of being quickly and easily administered (Figure 1-2 and Figure 1-3). These usually do not require dosage calculations. They have the disadvantage of being expensive. If less than the premeasured dose is given, the balance of the syringe must be wasted because a used syringe is inappropriate for storage or reuse with another patient (Figure 1-4).

Ampules are small, single-dose containers with a breakable glass top. They are opened by breaking the glass top off. The clinician then inserts a

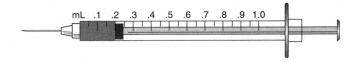

Figure 1-2 1 ml Syringe

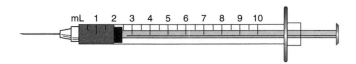

Figure 1-3 10 ml Syringe

sterile syringe and withdraws the medication. Ampules have the advantage of being single-dose units, which are relatively inexpensive and easy to store. The disadvantage of an ampule is that it must be handled carefully by the clinician to avoid minor self-inflicted lacerations.

Vials are glass containers with a rubber stopper (Figure 1-5). These may be single-dose containers or may allow multiple doses to be safely withdrawn when needed. The rubber stopper protects the contents from spilling and allows sterile technique to be used while the clinician withdraws medication. Each dose is drawn from the vial with a new sterile syringe. Vials are relatively inexpensive and allow a large range of doses. The disadvantage is that a large vial that is used infrequently may exceed its shelf life and become outdated.

A few medications are supplied as powders. These may be injected or orally administered. If the medication is injected, it must first be mixed with a liquid to form a solution. Medications that are supplied as a powder usually have a very short shelf life when in solution. They are supplied in a powder so they may be stored, without becoming impotent, until use.

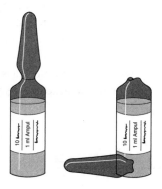

Figure 1-4 Ampule

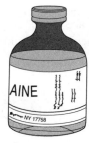

Figure 1-5 Vial

FACTORS INFLUENCING DOSAGE

Underlying Medical Conditions

Underlying medical conditions or pregnancy may **affect** the manner and dose of the medication administered.

Porphyria is an example of an underlying medical condition. It is a group of diseases in which patients must avoid barbiturates and alcohol. Another example is patients with chronic obstructive pulmonary disease (COPD), who may be dependent on catecholamines and should not receive beta-blocking medications, like propranolol or atenolol. Patients with liver diseases, such as cirrhosis, are unable to metabolize (break down) medications normally. Such people must be treated cautiously with any medication normally metabolized by the liver, such as lidocaine. Pregnancy creates special problems because many medications have undesired effects on the unborn fetus.

Patients with chronic medical conditions often take medication for their ailments. These medications and the possibility of interaction must be considered when giving other medications.

Age

Infants and children present special dosage problems. They are not simply small adults. Their chemistry is affected by adolescence, body proportion, and an inability to metabolize medications as effectively as adults.

Senior citizens also present special problems. They frequently have hydration problems, such as overhydration from congestive heart failure or moderate dehydration. They also may not metabolize medications as effectively as the typical adult.

Gender

A patient's gender has several influences on doses of medication. Males and females have body chemistry differences other than their sexual hormones. A female's hematocrit (concentration of red blood cells per unit of volume) and hemoglobin (amount of hemoglobin per unit of volume) measurements are lower than a male's. Men have a lower proportion of subcutaneous body fat than women. Men and women also have differences in the proportion of water volume per unit of body weight.

A woman's ability to receive medication is affected by pregnancy and considerations of how medication may affect the unborn fetus. The use of some medications by pregnant women may cause birth defects in their children.

The two sexual systems have specific disorders for which medication may be given.

Weight

Many medications have an effect on the body only within a specific concentration. To achieve a concentration of medication per unit of body water, the patient's body weight frequently serves as a guide to dosage determinations. Some medications are based on actual body weight. Others are based on the patient's ideal body weight. It is important to know which body weight is to be used to make the determination.

Medication is measured in metric units. Calculations related to body weight require body weight measurements in metric units also. It may be necessary to convert the patient's weight from pounds to kilograms.

Risk-Benefit Analysis

The administration of medication presents difficult choices. The possibility of **untoward effects**, **allergy**, and toxicity must be balanced against the patient's need for medication.

Cancer **chemotherapy** is a well-known example of risk-benefit analysis. One could question the wisdom of taking medication that causes violent vomiting, diarrhea, and hair loss. The benefit of chemotherapy is a desired cure for a disease that would otherwise cause death. In this example the risks are outweighed by the benefit.

The focal point of risk-benefit analysis is "Which presents a greater threat to the patient: the illness or injury or the potential negative effects of the medication?"

Which presents a greater threat to the patient: the illness, the injury, or the potential negative effects of treatment?

Exhibit 1-5 Risk-Benefit Question

Risk-benefit analysis depends on a thorough knowledge of pharmacokinetics and dosages. The USP and the PDR publish information about adverse reactions, interactions, etc. for this reason.

Tolerance

Tolerance is an individual's capacity to endure medication. Patients with high tolerance require higher doses of medication to achieve a therapeutic effect.

Patients with low tolerance require smaller doses to achieve a therapeutic effect. Patients with very low tolerance may suffer side effects, **hypersensitivity**, an allergic reaction, or **overdose** effects.

Tolerance may be acquired. **Acquired tolerance** develops as a result of the body adapting to the medication. As a patient adapts to a medication, larger doses are required to achieve the desired effect. Acquired tolerance is the first step toward **habituation**, the act of becoming accustomed to medication from frequent use.

A habituated drug user may be dependent or addicted. **Dependence** is a condition in which the user depends on the medication for his psychological well-being but is not physically addicted.

Addiction, by contrast, is a condition in which the user has physically adapted to the use of the medication and has acquired tolerance. Continued use of the medication is required to maintain physical well-being. Without continued doses of the drug, **withdrawal** symptoms will occur as the body systems adapt to the absence of the drug. Sudden cessation of drug use, known to some as "quitting cold turkey," may result in death. Rapidly acquired tolerance is a warning sign of potential addiction.

Drug potentiation can be a major factor in administration of medications. **Potentiation** is a dramatic increase in effect when two or more medications are used at the same time (**concomitantly**) by a patient. The increase in effect is greater than the sum of the medications' individual effects, if taken separately.

Potentiation can be beneficial by allowing two or more medications to be given concomitantly to achieve a desired effect. The same effect would normally require a larger dose of either medication given individually.

Potentiation can be damaging. The effect of multiple medications may increase beyond expected levels and become **toxic** or lead to behavioral toxicity. A common example is using alcohol while taking medication. Alcohol is a central-nervous-system-depressing drug. It should not be used with other central-nervous-system-depressing drugs, such as tranquilizers, sleeping medications, and some muscle relaxants.

The effects of combining medication(s) and alcohol can be dangerous.

Exhibit 1-6 Behavioral Toxicity

Synergism is related to potentiation. It is the harmonious action of two agents, not necessarily two medications. One of the agents may be an organ or system or even electricity. Together these agents produce an effect greater than or different from the added effects of both agents taken separately.

> Synergy means behavior of whole systems unpredicted by the behavior of their parts.
>
> —Richard Buckminster Fuller.

Exhibit 1-7 Synergy

Behavioral toxicity describes behavior that is detrimental to the patient's well-being. A patient under the influence of an hallucinogen may believe he can fly and jump from a tall building, a toxic behavior, because of that belief.

ROUTE OF ADMINISTRATION

Parenteral

A route of administration for medication by any means other than the gastrointestinal tract is a **parenteral** route. These include all forms of injection and adsorption.

Subcutaneous Injection

A **subcutaneous** injection is an injection given into the fat or connective tissue just beneath the skin. The **rate** of adsorption from this tissue into central circulation is slow. It is the most common route for medications that must be adsorbed over a period of time. Subcutaneous injections are usually limited to a volume of 1 ml or less. Common sites for subcutaneous injection include the superficial deltoid region of the arm and the abdominal area. Tetanus toxoid, epinephrine, allergy desensitization medication, and insulin are all commonly given as subcutaneous medications.

Intradermal

Intradermal (or intracutaneous) injections are given into a layer of the skin. This is commonly used to test for reactions, such as with the tuberculosis skin test or in allergy sensitivity testing. Common sites include the skin of the back or arms.

Intramuscular Injection

An **intramuscular** injection is an injection into the muscle. The rate of adsorption of medication from a muscle into the central circulation may vary from minutes to hours. Intramuscular medication is adsorbed more quickly than subcutaneous medication, but it is not as fast acting as an intravenous injection.

An intramuscular injection may be up to 5 ml of solution. The deltoid and the upper outer quadrant of the gluteus maximus are the most common sites for intramuscular injection. The anterior thigh is a common intramuscular injection site in children.

Intravenous Injection or Infusion

The **intravenous** (IV) route of injection or infusion uses direct access to the venous bloodstream. It has several advantages over other injection routes.

The rate of adsorption into central circulation is almost immediate. To be absorbed, intramuscular and subcutaneous injections depend on adequate perfusion. If perfusion is poor, they will not be effectively adsorbed until perfusion is restored.

The intravenous route may be used to replace fluid or blood volume. It may also be used to continuously administer medication over an extended period of time, with great control over the rate of administration.

Adsorption of medication by intramuscular and subcutaneous routes cannot be as effectively controlled as the IV route. These routes are also limited in the amount of medication that can be given.

Intraosseous Infusion

Intraosseous infusion is a technique of infusing medication directly into the bone marrow of a patient's long bone. This technique provides rapid vascular access in a critically injured infant or child. It is not considered a replacement for intravenous access but is reserved for emergencies. Medications that are commonly infused via the intraosseous route include atropine, dextrose, epinephrine, lidocaine, Ringer's lactate, and saline. There are no known medications that are absolutely contraindicated for intraosseous use at this time, but hypertonic solutions should be avoided because of the increased risk of osteomyelitis.

Intracardiac Injection

An **intracardiac** injection is an injection of medication directly into a chamber of the heart. This route of administration has no advantages over intravenous or endotracheal instillation. Intracardiac injection has several risks. These risks include injection into the muscle wall instead of into the chamber of the heart, laceration of a coronary artery, puncture of a lung, and interruption of cardiopulmonary resuscitation. For these reasons, it is no longer a popular route of administration.

Topical

Topical adsorption through the skin (**percutaneous**) or mucus membranes is a common route of administration. Some medications and many toxins can be adsorbed directly through the skin. Nitroglycerine paste or pads are examples of topical administration.

Mucosal

A mucus membrane frequently used is the area under the tongue. This is the **sublingual** route. It is used to administer nitroglycerine. It results in rapid adsorption directly into the circulatory system. Another mucus area is the eyes. Eyedrops are adsorbed through the **mucosa** of the eyes. Nose drops and nasal aerosols are also adsorbed through mucus membranes.

Inhalation

Inhalation is used for aerosol medications given to patients with lung disease or difficulty breathing. The most commonly administered medication, oxygen, is administered by inhalation.

Endotracheal Instillation

Endotracheal instillation is a technique of administering medication through an endotracheal tube into the mucosal membrane of a patient's lungs. An endotracheal tube is a sterile tube introduced into the mouth that reaches down the trachea into the main bronchus of the lungs. Medication administered by this route is rapidly adsorbed by the mucosa of the bronchi. This route is used in cardiac arrest emergencies when intravenous access is delayed. A popular mnemonic—NAVEL—is a reminder of five medications commonly administered through this route. It stands for naloxone (Narcan®), atropine, Valium, epinephrine, and lidocaine.

Nonparenteral

Nonparenteral routes of administration are through the alimentary canal. The alimentary canal is the digestive tract, which begins at the mouth and ends at the rectum. Nonparenteral medications are taken orally or rectally. These include suppositories, pills, caplets, gel caps, **elixirs**, and liquids, such as cough medicine or nose sprays.

Rectal **suppositories**, or rectal administration by soft catheter, are given for patients with active vomiting or rectal or lower gastrointestinal ailments, such as acute constipation. They are also given to pediatric patients who will not accept oral medication. Suppositories are commonly prescribed for patients who are vomiting and are unable to take or keep down oral medication. Some suppositories may be administered vaginally.

Medications given through the digestive tract are painlessly and easily taken. These medications are commonly prescribed for patients to take at home. A disadvantage of oral medicines is the first pass effect.

FIRST PASS EFFECT

The **first pass effect** is one of several ways the body metabolizes medication. The digestive tract has a circulatory pathway, or portal circulation, of blood from the digestive organs into the liver. The liver metabolizes foreign substances in the bloodstream. The cleaned-up blood passes out of the liver through the hepatic vein into the inferior vena cava. Orally administered medications are partially metabolized by the liver in the first pass through the portal circulation, before they pass through the rest of the body. This reduces, but does not completely eliminate, medications' effectiveness. The first pass effect must be considered when determining doses of oral medicines.

Additional disadvantages to accurate dosing occur when liver (hepatic) function is impaired. A normal dose, usually reduced by the first pass effect, may unexpectedly be excessive. Medication may not metabolize, as normally expected, by the first pass effect through the portal circulation because of a patient's liver failure. The medication builds up in the blood stream and may quickly approach overdose concentration.

BLOOD BRAIN BARRIER

The blood brain barrier, also known as the "hematoencephalic barrier," is a delicate membrane lining blood vessels in the brain. It separates nerve tissue of the brain from the circulatory system. It partially insulates the brain from damaging chemicals in the blood and helps control body regulatory mechanisms. Some medications diffuse across this barrier.

Antihistamines, for example, may be taken for sinus congestion and headaches. Most antihistamines cross the blood brain barrier and induce drowsiness. If drowsiness is not desired (an untoward effect), an antihistamine that doesn't cross the barrier would be more effective.

DOSAGE

A dose of medication is the quantity to be administered at one time. A **therapeutic** dose is an amount that will produce the effects for which it is given. A quantity too small to produce the desired effect is subtherapeutic, or below therapeutic levels. A quantity that is too large and produces undesired effects is supratherapeutic and is an overdose. Overdoses that produce deleterious effects are toxic. A lethal overdose results in death.

A loading dose is an initial dose intended to establish therapeutic levels of medication. Maintenance doses maintain the therapeutic level but are generally smaller than the loading dose. A therapeutic hiatus is a drop in the medication level to a concentration below a therapeutic level. This occurs when a loading dose is not properly followed with maintenance doses.

THERAPEUTIC ENVELOPE

The **therapeutic envelope** is a range of dosages, from the smallest effective dose to the strongest effective dose, within which a medication has a beneficial effect on the patient (Figure 1-6).

INFECTIOUS DISEASES

Infectious diseases may be transmitted between health care provider and patient. The risk of contracting an infectious disease is manageable and may be reduced to a very minimal risk.

The disease of greatest concern may be acquired immunodeficiency syndrome (AIDS). This disease is caused by the human immunodeficiency virus (HIV). Other diseases, such as tuberculosis, are also dangerous and opportunistic infections. Many AIDS patients have asymptomatic tuberculosis.

HIV is transmitted through sexual contact, exposure to infected blood or blood components, and perinatally from mother to neonate. HIV has been

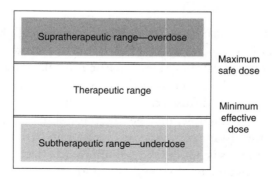

Figure 1-6 Therapeutic Envelope

isolated from blood, semen, vaginal secretions, saliva, tears, breast milk, cerebrospinal fluid, amniotic fluid, and urine and is likely to be isolated from other body fluids, secretions, and excretions. However, epidemiologic evidence has implicated only blood, semen, vaginal secretions, and possibly breast milk in transmission.[8]

The U.S. Department of Health and Human Services has a division entitled the Centers for Disease Control and Prevention. The Centers for Disease Control and Prevention is frequently called the CDC.

The CDC has published in the *Morbidity and Mortality Weekly Report* "Recommendations for the Prevention of HIV Transmission in Health Care Settings."[9] Compliance with these recommendations will protect the provider against all other infectious diseases transmitted through body fluids. (Please refer to Exhibit 1-8.)

Health care workers are continually exposed to patients with infectious diseases. An exposure with a high probability of causing infection is a significant exposure.

The significance of an exposure depends on the manner in which the disease is communicated and the type of exposure. For example, a health care worker who has an immunity from a childhood exposure to chicken pox is exposed to a child with chicken pox. This exposure is not significant because the worker has a preexisting immunity to the disease.

Many serious diseases, including AIDS and hepatitis B, are blood borne. Blood-borne diseases require an exposure of body fluids—such as semen, vaginal secretions, breast milk, or blood—to contact a person's body fluids or mucus membranes for the disease to be communicated. Blood-borne diseases may be transmitted sexually. Significant exposures to blood-borne diseases can occur as listed in Exhibit 1-9 on page 27. The risk of hepatitis B being contracted during exposure to a patient's blood is high. This risk can be almost completely eliminated by administration of the antihepatitis B vaccine before potential exposure. Professional health care providers are unwise and may present a risk of infection to others if they fail to take advantage of this excellent vaccine.

---

[8] U.S. Department of Health and Human Services, Centers for Disease Control. (1988, June 24). Update to Universal Precautions for Prevention of Transmission of Human Immunodeficiency Virus, Hepatitis B Virus, and Other Blood Borne Pathogens in Health Care Settings. *Morbidity and Mortality Weekly Report, 37*(24).

[9] U.S. Department of Health and Human Services, Centers for Disease Control. (1987, August 21). Recommendations for Prevention of HIV Transmission in Health Care Settings. *Morbidity and Mortality Weekly Report, 36*(2S).

1. Take care to prevent injuries when using needles, scalpels, and other sharp instruments or devices; when handling sharp instruments after procedures; when cleaning used instruments; and when disposing of used needles. Do not recap used needles by hand; do not remove used needles from disposable syringes by hand; and do not bend, break, or otherwise manipulate used needles by hand. Place used disposable syringes and needles, scalpel blades, and other sharp items in puncture-resistant containers for disposal. Locate the puncture-resistant containers as close to the use area as is practical.
2. Use protective barriers to prevent exposure to blood, body fluids containing visible blood, and other fluids to which universal precautions apply. The type of protective barrier(s) should be appropriate for the procedure being performed and the type of exposure anticipated.
3. Immediately and thoroughly wash hands and other skin surfaces that are contaminated with blood, body fluids containing visible blood, or other body fluids to which universal precautions apply.

Glove Use for Phlebotomy

Gloves should always be available to health care workers who wish to use them for phlebotomy. In addition, the following general guidelines apply:

1. Use gloves for performing phlebotomy when the health-care worker has cuts, scratches, or other breaks in his/her skin.
2. Use gloves in situations where the health-care worker judges that hand contamination with blood may occur—for example, when performing phlebotomy on an uncooperative patient.
3. Use gloves for performing finger and/or heel sticks on infants and children.
4. Use gloves when persons are receiving training in phlebotomy.

The following general guidelines are recommended for the selection of gloves:

1. Use sterile gloves for procedures involving contact with normally sterile areas of the body.
2. Use examination gloves for procedures involving contact with mucous membranes, unless otherwise indicated, and for other patient care or diagnostic procedures that do not require the use of sterile gloves.
3. Change gloves between patient contacts.
4. Do not wash or disinfect surgical or examination gloves for reuse. Washing with surfactants may cause "wicking"—i.e., the enhanced penetration of liquids through undetected holes in the glove. Disinfecting agents may cause deterioration.
5. Use general-purpose utility gloves (e.g., rubber household gloves) for housekeeping chores involving potential blood contact and for instrument cleaning and decontamination procedures. Utility gloves may be decontaminated and reused but should be discarded if they are peeling, cracked, or discolored, or if they have punctures, tears, or other evidence of deterioration.

Adapted from: U.S. Federal Health and Human Services, Centers for Disease Control and Prevention. *Morbidity and Mortality Weekly Report*, June 24 and August 21, 1988.

Exhibit 1-8 Universal Precautions

Significant exposure varies depending on the substance to which the exposure is made. Chemicals and some diseases may be atmospherically spread or absorbed through the skin. For the purposes of blood-borne pathogens significant exposure is defined by the Centers for Disease Control and Prevention as:

An "exposure" that may place a Health Care Worker (HCW) at risk for Human Immunodeficiency Virus (HIV) infection and therefore requires consideration of PPE [Personal Protective Equipment] is defined as a percutaneous injury (e.g., a needle stick or cut with a sharp object), contact of mucous membrane or nonintact skin (e.g., when the exposed skin is chapped, abraded, or afflicted with dermatitis), or contact with intact skin when the duration of contact is prolonged (i.e., several minutes or more) or involves an extensive area with blood, tissue, or other body fluids. Body fluids include (a) semen, vaginal secretions, or other body fluids contaminated with visible blood that have been implicated in the transmission of HIV infection; and (b) cerebrospinal, synovial, pleural, peritoneal, pericardial, and amniotic fluids, which have an undetermined risk for transmitting HIV. In addition, any direct contact (i.e., without barrier protection) to concentrated HIV in a research laboratory or production facility is considered an "exposure" that requires clinical evaluation and consideration of the need for PPE.

Source: Florida Department of Health and Rehabilitative Services, Office of Emergency Medical Services. Program Letter 88–20, October 18, 1988.

Exhibit 1-9 More Universal Precautions

MEDICALERT

Some patients wear a **MedicAlert** tag. MedicAlert is a private nonprofit organization that provides bracelets or pendants for sale to patients who have significant medical conditions. Wearing a MedicAlert tag provides important information about a patient's medical condition or allergy when he is unconscious or otherwise unable to communicate. Always check for MedicAlert tags before administering medication to an unconscious patient in an emergency setting. MedicAlert tags may be purchased at most pharmacies. The organization's Web site is http://www.medicalert.org/home/Homegradient.aspx.

Do not believe in anything simply because you have heard it. Do not believe in anything simply because it is spoken and rumored by many. Do not believe in anything simply because it is found written in your religious books. Do not believe in anything merely on the authority of your teachers and elders. Do not believe in traditions because they have been handed down for many generations. But after observation and analysis, when you find that anything agrees with reason and is conducive to the good and benefit of one and all, then accept it and live up to it.

—Buddha.

Exhibit 1-10

Chapter 2

Ratio Equations

> You cannot teach a man anything.
>
> You can only help him discover it within himself.
>
> —Galileo.

Exhibit 2-1

OBJECTIVES

Upon completion of this chapter the clinician should be able to:

1. Identify and use ratios
2. Explain why intuitive operations should be practiced with equations
3. Identify and use integer factors
4. Identify and use non-integer factors
5. Explain and use correct order of operations in solving equations
6. Solve simple algebraic equations for *x*

KEY TERMS

denominator	order of operations
division	product
equation	proportion
factor	ratio
fraction	reciprocal
integer	unknown
multiplication	whole number
numerator	

RATIOS

Why use ratios when there is a common sense answer to your question that I can do in my head? **Ratios** are important to setting up **equations**. The clinician may be able and strongly tempted to solve these simple problems early in the text without using the ratio/equation set-up process. Go ahead and figure out the common sense answer. Then go back and set up the equation. When word problems get more complex, the skills learned by practicing with the simple ratios here will help the clinician set up equations for these more complicated operations. So it is wise to resist going intuitively to the answer and skipping the set-up process. Later the answers will not be intuitive, and if you skip the set-up process now, you will have lost a tool you need to solve more complex problems. The purpose of these problems is to get you to begin to recognize the set-up process. Calculation of dosages is fairly simple and straightforward. It will become confusing when conversions between units such as volume to mass are given over periods of time or calculations are based on patient weight. As you become more experienced, you will learn to take shortcuts, and that is one advantage of experience.

A ratio is a constant relationship between two values. We deal with ratios every day. These include prices, such as a ratio of money to gallons of milk, or time, such as the number of hours per work shift. Ratios are used to calculate related values, such as costs or amounts of medication to administer.

Ratios may be written with a colon: 8 hours:1 shift

or as a fraction: $\dfrac{8 \text{ hours}}{1 \text{ shift}}$

Exhibit 2-2 Ratio Equations

When the expression contains a colon, it is read as 8 hours *to* 1 shift. When it is written with a fraction line, it is read as 8 hours *per* 1 shift. The form using a fraction line is preferred for dosage calculations. Some familiar ratios appear in Exhibit 2-3.

---

60 minutes/hour	60 min:1 hour
7 days/week	7 days:1 week
12 eggs/dozen	12 eggs:1 dozen
2 shoes/pair	2 shoes:1 pair

Exhibit 2-3 Common Ratios

A ratio is a constant relation **proportion**. *Constant* means the relation between the two values does not change. For each 1 dozen eggs there are 12 eggs, and for each hour of the day there are 60 minutes. It also means that for every part of 1 dozen eggs there is an exact (related) same part of 12 eggs. Similarly, it means that for every part of an hour there is an exact (related) same part of 60 minutes. One half of 1 dozen eggs is equal to one half of 12 eggs because 1 dozen eggs is related to 12 eggs.

If: 1 dozen eggs is equal to 12 eggs

Then: $\frac{1}{2}$(1 dozen eggs) is equal to $\frac{1}{2}$(12 eggs)

Exhibit 2-4 Example Ratio Problem

If asked how many eggs are in one half dozen, a person can quickly answer, "There are 6." This problem is easily solved intuitively without using paper and pencil. However, ratios are used to set up mathematical expressions called equations. Using an equation provides the clinician an organized approach to solving problems.

This is useful for problems more complex than "How many eggs are in one half dozen?"

Setting up a problem as an equation gives the clinician an organized mathematical approach to problem solving.

Exhibit 2-5 Setting Up Equations

This approach will work with all dosage calculation problems. During this course of study, intuitively solve those problems that seem simple. Then set up and solve them in a ratio equation. This will provide practice with equations. Solving problems intuitively without learning the skills of using equations will leave the clinician unprepared when difficult problems are encountered.

An equation is a mathematical expression that contains an equal sign (=) and two parts, one on each side of the equal sign. Each side of an equation is equal to the other.

The advantage of using an equation is that if one side is known, then the other side (which is not known) can be calculated. A clinician can manipulate an equation by adding, subtracting, multiplying, or dividing both sides without changing its value or the correct answer.

> A clinician can add, subtract, multiply, or divide both sides of an equation without changing its value or the correct answer.

Exhibit 2-6 Solving Equations

In Exhibit 2-7, both sides are divided by 3 to solve the equation and get all known and **integer** information on the one side and all the **unknown** on the other side.

Problem: $3x = 6$

Objective: Get x alone on one side of the equation so that the other side is equal to x.

Solution: To get $3x$ alone (to be $1x$), it is divided by the integer 3.

The same operation must be performed on both sides, or the equation will have been incorrectly changed.

$3x = 6$

$3x \div 3 = 6 \div 3$

$1x = 2$

Exhibit 2-7 Example Equation

It doesn't matter which side has the known information. A clinician may work left to right or vice versa. In Exhibit 2-7, an arbitrary choice was made to work from left to right. The equation could have been solved in the same manner from right to left, as in Exhibit 2-8.

Problem: $6 = 3x$

$6 = 3x$

$6 \div 3 = 3x \div 3$

$2 = 1x$

Exhibit 2-8 Example Equation

In Exhibit 2-9, both sides are multiplied by 2 to solve the equation.

Problem: $^1/_2 x = 3$

Objective: Get x alone on one side of the equation so that the other side is equal to x.

Solution: To get $^1/_2 x$ alone (to be $1x$), it is multiplied by the integer 2.

The same operation must be performed on both sides, or the equation will have been incorrectly changed.

$^1/_2 x = 3$

$^1/_2 x * 2 = 3 * 2$

$1x = 6$

Exhibit 2-9 Example Equation

In Exhibit 2-10, both sides have 2 added to solve the equation.

Problem: $x - 2 = 4$

Remember that x is the same as $1x$.

Objective: Get x alone on one side of the equation so that the other side is equal to x (or $1x$).

Solution: To get $x - 2$ alone (to be $1x$), the integer 2 must be added to both sides.

The same operation must be performed on both sides, or the equation will have been incorrectly changed.

$x - 2 = 4$

$x - 2 + 2 = 4 + 2$

$1x = 6$

Exhibit 2-10 Example Equation

In Exhibit 2-11, the equation is solved much like Exhibit 2-10, except that both sides have 2 subtracted (instead of added) to solve the equation.

Problem: $x + 2 = 4$

Objective: Get x alone on one side of the equation so that the other side is equal to x.

Solution: To get $x + 2$ alone (to be $1x$), subtract 2 from both sides.

The same operation must be performed on both sides, or the equation will have been incorrectly changed.

$1x + 2 = 4$

$1x + 2 - 2 = 4 - 2$

$1x = 2$

Exhibit 2-11 Example Equation

FACTORS

A **factor** is a number or expression that may be multiplied by another factor to give a mathematical expression. In the mathematical expression 6, factors multiplied by each other to yield 6 may be [1 * 6] or [2 * 3] or [1.5 * 4]

Expression	Factors
6	1 * 6
	2 * 3
	1.5 * 4

In the expression *24 hours* there are several factors. Factors are not always **whole numbers**. They are sometimes words, such as *hours*. These non-number factors are non-integer factors. For simplicity non-integer factors are called "word factors."

Expression	Factors
24 hours	1 * 24 * hours
	2 * 12 * hours
	3 * 8 * hours
	4 * 6 * hours

A word factor that has no expressed integer always has an implied integer value of 1 (Exhibit 2-12).

x is the same as 1x

hour is the same as 1 hour

ml is the same as 1 ml

60 minutes/hour is the same as 60 minutes/1 hour

ml/60 drops is the same as 1 ml/60 drops

Exhibit 2-12 Factors

A word factor (such as the word *hour*) is used in arithmetic operations like a number. **Multiplication** and **division** by word factors may be performed on any number or expression. To multiply by a word factor, place it in the numerator. To divide by a word factor, place it in the denominator.

The **numerator** is the top number in a **fraction** and the number to be divided. The **denominator** is the bottom number of a fraction and the number of parts by which the numerator is divided.

Addition and subtraction can only be conducted with expressions that have similar word factors. For example, one cannot subtract 4 apples from 6 oranges. One can only subtract a number of apples from another number of apples and a number of oranges from another number of oranges. Please refer to Exhibit 2-13 for instructions and Exhibit 2-14 for an example equation.

Word factors are not changed by arithmetic operations unless the arithmetic operation uses another word factor. When an arithmetic operation is performed, the number factor may be changed, but not the word factor. A word factor in the denominator will remain there, and a word factor in the numerator will remain there.

To multiply by a word factor, place it in the numerator.
To divide by a word factor, place it in the denominator.

Addition and subtraction can only be conducted with expressions that have the same word factors.

Exhibit 2-13 Working with Word Factors

Problem: $x = 24$ hours $- 8$ hours

Objective: Get x alone on one side of the equation so that the other side is equal to x.

Solution: To solve for x, subtract 8 hours from 24 hours.

The operation is indicated only for one side of the equation and is not a change in the equation.

$x = 24$ hours $- 8$ hours

$x = 24$ hours
$\underline{- 8\text{ hours}}$
16 hours

$x = 16$ hours

Exhibit 2-14 Example Equation

Word factors may be changed by arithmetic operations that use word factors. When a word factor is divided by another word factor, the answer is a new expression, but not a new number. Division of a word factor by another factor must be written out. If you wished to divide 8 hours by 1 shift, the expression would be written as shown in Exhibit 2-16.

Problem: $x = 24$ hours/8 hours

Objective: Get x alone on one side of the equation so that the other side is equal to x.

Solution: To solve for x, divide 24 hours by 8 hours as indicated.

The operation is indicated only for one side of the equation and is not a change in the equation.

$$x = \frac{24 \text{ hours}}{8 \text{ hours}}$$

In this example, the factor of hours is divided by hours.
Anything divided by itself is equal to 1.

$$x = \frac{24 \text{ hours}}{8 \text{ hours}}$$

$$x = \frac{24 * 1}{8 * 1}$$ This leaves only
the numerical
factors to solve.

$x = 3$

Exhibit 2-15 Example Equation

$$\frac{8 \text{ hours}}{\text{shift}} \text{ (or 8 hours:shift)}$$

This would be reported as 8 hours *per* shift.

Exhibit 2-16 Example Ratio

In a fraction, any number divided by itself is equal to the integer 1. This is also true of word factors.

Any factor (integer or word) divided by itself equals 1.

Exhibit 2-17 Factors

Equations should always be simplified by completing any arithmetic functions indicated. The arithmetic function indicated in Exhibit 2-18 is on the right side and is a multiplication of $^{1}/_{2}$ times 12 eggs. This requires the multiplication of a fraction factor ($^{1}/_{2}$), a whole number factor (12), and a word factor (eggs).

$$x = {}^{1}/_{2} \text{ (12 eggs)}$$

Exhibit 2-18 Example Equation

A whole number is the same as a fraction of itself with a denominator of 1. To multiply a fraction and a whole number, multiply the numerator times the numerator and the denominator times the denominator, as in Exhibit 2-19.

The word factor *eggs* will not work in an arithmetic problem, but it cannot just be ignored for convenience. It must be carried through the equation and written out everywhere the factor (eggs) should be in the arithmetic problem. To work the problem of $^{1}/_{2}$ (12 eggs), multiply as shown in Exhibit 2-19.

Step 1: Convert the whole number and word factor to fractions.	$12 \text{ eggs} = \dfrac{12}{1} \text{ eggs} = \dfrac{12 * \text{eggs}}{1 * 1}$
Step 2: Multiply the fractions (numerators * numerators and denominators * denominators).	$x = \dfrac{1}{2} * \dfrac{12}{1} * \dfrac{\text{eggs}}{1}$
The answer is derived, but it is not completely simplified.	$x = \dfrac{1 * 12 * \text{eggs}}{2 * 1 * 1}$
	$x = \dfrac{12 \text{ eggs}}{2}$
Step 3: Recall that any thing over 1 is a whole expression.	$x = \dfrac{6 \text{ eggs}}{1} = 6 \text{ eggs}$

Exhibit 2-19 Example Equation

ORDER OF OPERATIONS

In the previous examples both multiplication and division were required to solve for x. Sometimes solving for the unknown requires multiple operations. The correct answer of a problem depends on the order in which the operations are performed. Exhibit 2-20 illustrates this.

In the operation $x = 5 + 5 * 10$

If the addition is performed first,

the outcome is:

$x = (5 + 5) * 10$

$x = 10 * 10$

$x = 100$

If the multiplication is performed first, the outcome is:

$x = 5 + (5 * 10)$

$x = 5 + 50$

$x = 55$

So the order of operations clearly makes a difference!

Exhibit 2-20 Order of Operations Example

The standard **order of operations** for mathematical operations follows these rules:

1. Always solve from inside to outside of parentheses.
2. Exponent operations are performed first.
3. Multiplication or division is second. There is no preferred order of operations between these two.
4. Addition or subtraction is performed last. There is no preferred order between these two.

In Exhibit 2-21, it is necessary to divide and to multiply. There is no preferred order between multiplication and division. x represents the unknown factor. Factor the equation to get x alone. The expression that remains on the other side of the equal (=) sign is the solution.

First, multiply both sides by the denominator of x to convert x to a whole expression rather than a fraction	$\dfrac{3x}{2} = 30$
	$\dfrac{2 * 3x}{2} = 30 * 2$
	$3x = 60$
Second, divide both sides by the factor of x to get x alone as $1x$	$3x \div 3 = 60 \div 3$
	$x = 20$

Exhibit 2-21 Order of Operations Example

RECIPROCAL NUMBERS

In Exhibit 2-21, both sides of the equation were multiplied and then divided to obtain x with a factor of 1. This may also be done in one operation by multiplying by a fraction.

Every expression other than zero has a matching expression by which it can be multiplied to give a **product** of 1. This matching expression is the **reciprocal**. See Exhibit 2-22 for examples and Exhibit 2-23 for a sample equation.

Expression	*	Reciprocal	=	Product
$\dfrac{1}{2}$	*	$\dfrac{2}{1}$	=	$\dfrac{2}{2} = 1$
$\dfrac{1}{4}$	*	$\dfrac{4}{1}$	=	$\dfrac{4}{4} = 1$
$\dfrac{4\ ml}{1\ min}$	*	$\dfrac{1\ min}{4\ ml}$	=	$\dfrac{4\ ml\ min}{4\ ml\ min} = 1$

Exhibit 2-22 Reciprocal Numbers

$\dfrac{3x}{2} = 30$ — Identify the reciprocal number of x and then go to step 2.

$\dfrac{3x}{2} * \dfrac{2}{3} = \dfrac{30}{1} * \dfrac{2}{3}$ — Multiply both sides by the reciprocal of x (which is $2/3$) to get $1x$ alone.

$\dfrac{3x * 2}{2 * 3} = \dfrac{30 * 2}{1 * 3}$

$\dfrac{6x}{6} = \dfrac{60}{3}$ — Simplify the fraction.

$x = 20$

Exhibit 2-23 Reciprocal Number Example

It is important to accurately identify whether word factors are in the numerator or denominator. In 4 ml/minute, *ml* is in the numerator, and *minute* is in the denominator. The denominator of any whole expression is always 1.

Any word factor divided by itself yields a product of 1. The reciprocal of an expression containing a word factor will have a matching word factor in the inverse location.

To factor an expression to 1 in a combined operation:

1. Identify the factor of x.

2. Identify the reciprocal of the factor of x.

3. Multiply both sides of the equation by the reciprocal of the factor of x.

Exhibit 2-24 Using Reciprocal Numbers

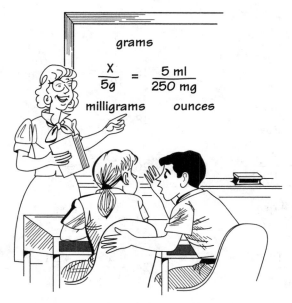

"Hey, isn't this algebra
or something?"

Figure 2-1 Algebra

REVIEW PROBLEMS

Solve the following ratio equations for x.

1. $\dfrac{4x}{2} = 30$

2. $\dfrac{4x}{2} = \dfrac{60}{2}$

3. $\dfrac{2x}{4} = \dfrac{15}{2}$

4. $\dfrac{x}{2} = \dfrac{15}{2}$

5. $\dfrac{x}{4} = 5$

6. $\dfrac{x}{4} = \dfrac{5}{2}$

7. $\dfrac{x}{2} = \dfrac{10}{5}$

8. $\dfrac{x}{3} = \dfrac{10}{5}$

9. $\dfrac{x}{4} = \dfrac{10}{5}$

10. $\dfrac{x}{2} = \dfrac{5}{10}$

11. $\dfrac{x}{3} = \dfrac{5}{10}$

12. $\dfrac{x}{4} = \dfrac{5}{10}$

13. $\dfrac{x}{4} = \dfrac{4}{1}$

14. $\dfrac{2x}{3} = \dfrac{2}{3}$

15. $\dfrac{3x}{2} = \dfrac{2}{3}$

16. $\dfrac{x}{100} = \dfrac{1 \text{ quarter}}{25}$

17. $\dfrac{2x}{50¢} = \dfrac{1 \text{ quarter}}{25¢}$

18. $\dfrac{x}{1 \text{ gal}} = \dfrac{4 \text{ qt}}{1 \text{ gal}}$

19. $\dfrac{x}{0.5 \text{ gal}} = \dfrac{4 \text{ qt}}{1 \text{ gal}}$

20. $\dfrac{2x}{1 \text{ gal}} = \dfrac{4 \text{ qt}}{1 \text{ gal}}$

21. $\dfrac{4x}{1 \text{ gal}} = \dfrac{4 \text{ qt}}{1 \text{ gal}}$

22. $\dfrac{x}{12} = \dfrac{1 \text{ case}}{24}$

23. $\dfrac{x}{1 \text{ case}} = \dfrac{12}{24}$

24. $\dfrac{x}{4 \text{ mg}} = \dfrac{4 \text{ ml}}{1 \text{ mg}}$

25. $\dfrac{x}{4 \text{ mg}} = \dfrac{5 \text{ ml}}{10 \text{ mg}}$

26. $2 \text{ ml } x = 30 \text{ mg}$

27. $2 \text{ mg } x = 30 \text{ ml}$

28. $2x = \dfrac{15 \text{ mg}}{30 \text{ ml}}$

29. $2x = \dfrac{15 \text{ ml}}{30 \text{ mg}}$

30. $\dfrac{x}{2 \text{ ml}} = \dfrac{15 \text{ mg}}{30 \text{ ml}}$

31. $\dfrac{x}{2 \text{ mg}} = \dfrac{15 \text{ ml}}{30 \text{ mg}}$

32. $\dfrac{x}{15 \text{ ml}} = \dfrac{2 \text{ mg}}{30 \text{ mg}}$

33. $\dfrac{x}{10 \text{ ml}} = \dfrac{5 \text{ mg}}{10 \text{ ml}}$

34. $5x = 25 \text{ mg}$

35. $\dfrac{x}{10 \text{ L}} = \dfrac{2 \text{ mg}}{1 \text{ L}}$

36. $\dfrac{x}{10 \text{ L}} = \dfrac{1 \text{ mcg}}{1 \text{ L}}$

37. $\dfrac{x}{10 \text{ L}} = \dfrac{2g}{1 \text{ L}}$

38. $\dfrac{x}{10 \text{ L}} = \dfrac{1 \text{ mg}}{1 \text{ L}}$

39. $\dfrac{x}{5 \text{ L}} = \dfrac{1 \text{ g}}{1 \text{ L}}$

40. $\dfrac{x}{5 \text{ L}} = \dfrac{5 \text{ g}}{1 \text{ L}}$

41. $\dfrac{x}{1 \text{ L}} = \dfrac{1 \text{ g}}{5 \text{ L}}$

42. $\dfrac{x}{1 \text{ L}} = \dfrac{5 \text{ g}}{5 \text{ L}}$

43. $\dfrac{x}{2 \text{ L}} = \dfrac{2 \text{ g}}{4 \text{ L}}$

44. $\dfrac{x}{4 \text{ L}} = \dfrac{2 \text{ g}}{2 \text{ L}}$

45. $\dfrac{x}{2 \text{ g}} = \dfrac{2 \text{ L}}{4 \text{ L}}$

46. $\dfrac{x}{2 \text{ g}} = \dfrac{4 \text{ L}}{2 \text{ L}}$

47. $\dfrac{x}{2 \text{ g}} = \dfrac{2 \text{ ml}}{4 \text{ ml}}$

48. $\dfrac{x}{2 \text{ g}} = \dfrac{4 \text{ ml}}{2 \text{ ml}}$

49. $\dfrac{x}{2 \text{ L}} = \dfrac{2 \text{ g}}{4 \text{ g}}$

50. $\dfrac{x}{2 \text{ L}} = \dfrac{4 \text{ g}}{2 \text{ g}}$

Chapter 3

Metric System

You shall do no unrighteousness in judgment, in measure of length, in weight, or in quantity. Just balances, just weights, shall ye have.

—Leviticus. Chapter 19, verse 35–36.

Exhibit 3-1

OBJECTIVES

Upon completion of this chapter the clinician should be able to:

1. Distinguish between counting and measuring systems
2. Demonstrate a working knowledge of major units of measure in the metric system, including units of volume, mass, and length
3. Identify and explain metric prefixes
4. Use unit conversion factors to convert between different metric units
5. Demonstrate a working knowledge of major units of measure in the apothecary system
6. Use unit conversion factors to make conversions between basic metric and apothecary units

KEY TERMS

apothecary system
Arabic number system
Celsius
centi
deci
deka
gram
hecto
kilo
kilogram

liter
mega
meter
metric system
micro
milli
nano
syrup
unit conversion
  factor

SYSTEMS OF MEASUREMENT

The Industrial Revolution brought many changes to the world. A concept of standardizing machine parts was developed initially by the military organizations of the world. Until the advent of the Industrial Revolution, even simple machines were individually handcrafted without interchangeable parts. Industry recognized the need to have tools and weapons with interchangeable parts. It was costly to take machines out of service because a single part failed. Replacement of interchangeable spare parts by unskilled labor was a solution to the problem.

In the past, different areas of the world developed their own systems of measurement. The British developed the **apothecary system**, which the American colonies adopted. Americans still use many apothecary and household measurements. With the Industrial Revolution and increased world trade, the need for a system of common measures became clear. The British mile, the nautical mile, and the Roman mile are all different. The cubit, by which Noah measured his ark, bears small resemblance to the British yard or foot.

The U.S. legislature recognized this need for an international system of measure. In 1975, it passed the Metric Conversion Act, which says that the United States will convert to the **metric system**. The act does not set a specific time frame for conversion. Scientific units of measure are already universal and have led the way. Other units of measure will follow.

There exists in the United States three systems of measure: the metric system, the apothecary system, and the household system. They have units of measure that are approximately related to each other but are not exactly equal. This text will concentrate on the metric system because it is the primary system used in medical science.

THE METER

In 1799, the French Academy of Sciences convened to develop an international standard of measurement. Its members recognized that calculated astronomical measurements were the most precise measurements available to them. These scientists decided to use the calculated distance from the equator to the North Pole of the Earth as a starting measurement for a unit of length. To reduce that measurement to manageable size, they divided it by factors of 10 until they had a unit of length about the size of a man's stride. They found this division was one ten-millionth of the distance between the pole and the equator. They called this unit a **meter**, based on the Greek word for "measure." The metric system of measurement is built on the meter.

As the need for more precise measurements developed, the length of the meter was redefined. In 1983 the meter was defined as the length of the path traveled by light in a vacuum during an interval of 1/299,792,458 of a second.

A single unit of measure was not enough. Larger and smaller units needed to be defined. The **Arabic number system**, using 10 as a base, was accepted worldwide. The scientists reasoned that a measurement system using the base 10 would allow simple mathematical conversion between different units of measure. The meter was divided by 10, then by 10 again, and so on to form smaller units of measure. It was multiplied by 10, then by 10 again, and so on to form larger units. Each unit of measure was identified by a prefix indicating whether it was multiplied or divided and by how much, as shown on Table 3-1.

Table 3-1 Metric Prefixes

Multiplication Prefixes

mega	*	1,000,000
kilo	*	1,000
hecto	*	100
deka	*	10

Division Prefixes

deci	÷	10
centi	÷	100
milli	÷	1,000
micro	÷	1,000,000
nano	÷	1,000,000,000

A *kilo*meter is 1 meter multiplied by 1,000.
A *milli*meter is 1 meter divided by 1,000.

THE LITER

With units of length established, standard units of volume also were needed. The most universally available substance that could be shaped to any container or volume was distilled water. The scientists started with a cubic meter of water as a unit of measure and discovered it weighed about 220 pounds. This was not conveniently manageable. They reduced the cubic meter to a decimeter (one tenth of a meter) and discovered a very manageable unit of size and weight (about 2.2 lb). This was called the **liter**. Smaller and larger units of a liter are developed the same as the meter, using the same prefixes.

THE GRAM

Units of weight and units of volume are not related in the same way for every material. A milliliter of lead weighs a lot more than a milliliter of air. A standard metric relationship between weight and volume was established only for distilled water. A weight equivalent to a liter was too much for the desired starting point. The scientists settled on a weight of one milliliter of water as the unit of weight to be called the **gram**. Smaller and larger units of a gram are created in the same way as the meter and liter, using the same prefixes (Table 3-2).

Table 3-2 Metric Units

Units of measure—larger than the base unit			
Prefix	**Meter**	**Liter**	**Gram**	**Size of Unit**
mega-	megameter	megaliter	megagram	1,000,000
kilo-	kilometer	kiloliter	kilogram	1,000
hecto-	hectometer	hectoliter	hectogram	100
deka-	decameter	dekaliter	dekagram	10

Units of measure—smaller than the base unit			
Prefix	**Meter**	**Liter**	**Gram**	**Size of Unit**
deci-	decimeter	deciliter	decigram	.1
centi-	centimeter	centiliter	centigram	.01
milli-	millimeter	milliliter	milligram	.001
micro-	micrometer	microliter	microgram	.000001
nano-	nanometer	nanoliter	nanogram	.000000001

THE METRIC SYSTEM

The simplicity of the metric system is that all the units are sized up or down in the same way, using the same prefixes and using the base 10, as already established by our counting system.

In the metric system, known internationally as the International System of Units (ISU), there are seven basic units of measure, as listed in Table 3-3. All other metric units are derived from these basic units. For example, minutes are derived from seconds, hours from minutes, etc.

Table 3-3 International System of Units—Base Units

Quantity	Metric Unit	Symbol
length	meter	m
mass	kilogram	kg
temperature	degree Kelvin	°K
time	second	sec
electricity	ampere	a
luminous intensity	candle	c
amount of substance	mole	mol

Abbreviations of metric terms, as a general rule, use lowercase (not capitalized) letters, unless the metric term is derived from a proper name, as in the terms *Kelvin* or **Celsius**. An exception to this rule in this text is the abbreviation for the term *liter*. This text will use the uppercase letter *L* for liter to avoid possible confusion between the lowercase letter *l* and the numeral 1.

Table 3-4 lists a few metric units of measure derived from the ISU's seven basic units of measure.

Table 3-4 Additonal Units of Measure Derived from the ISU

Measure	Unit	Abbreviation
volume	liter	L
electrolyte concentration	milliequivalents	mEq
temperature	degree Celsius	°C
time	minute/hour/etc.	hr/min

METRIC CONVERSIONS

Conversions between larger or smaller units of metric measurements are easily calculated. There is a constant ratio between different units of measure. This ratio is used to make any desired conversions from one unit of measure to another. In Exhibit 3-2, to convert **kilograms** to grams, the ratio used is 1 kg/1,000 g. Any value of kilograms may be converted to an equivalent value of grams using this ratio in an equation.

Question: How many grams is 4.2 kg?

Solution: To solve for x, we can set up a ratio equation using the unit conversion factor for kilograms to grams.

$$\frac{x}{4.2 \text{ kg}} = \frac{1{,}000 \text{ g}}{1 \text{ kg}}$$

$$\frac{4.2 \text{ kg } (x)}{4.2 \text{ kg}} = \frac{(1{,}000 \text{ g}) \; 4.2 \text{ kg}}{1 \text{ kg}}$$

$$x = (1{,}000 \text{ g}) \; 4.2$$

$$x = 4{,}200 \text{ g}$$

Exhibit 3-2 Example Unit Conversion Factors

x was arbitrarily set up in the numerator on the left of this equation. x (the asked for and unknown number of grams) was related to the known number of kilograms (4.2 kg) as a ratio. The known standard metric ratio of grams to kilograms was used on the right of the equation. The ratio of grams to kilograms is known to be 1,000 g to 1 kg.

Grams were placed in the numerator on both sides of the equation. This is necessary to keep the equation in good form because kilograms was in the denominator on the left and should also be in the denominator on the right. The question asked for grams, so x represents a value in grams. x is easier to solve for if it is in the numerator.

UNIT CONVERSION FACTOR

A ratio may be used in an equation in any way that contributes to solving the equation. This means it may be used as:

$$1 \text{ kg}:1{,}000 \text{ g} \qquad \frac{1 \text{ kg}}{1{,}000 \text{ g}}$$

or as:

$$1{,}000 \text{ g}:1 \text{ kg} \qquad \frac{1{,}000 \text{ g}}{1 \text{ kg}}$$

This ratio is equal to the whole number 1 when it is reduced to its lowest terms. A ratio of an equal amount between two or more different units of measure equals 1 and is a **unit conversion factor**. This may be used to convert between different units of measure.

A unit conversion factor is a ratio of an equal amount of different units of measure. It is always equal to 1.

Exhibit 3-3 Unit Conversion Factor Definition

Any two units of like measure (volume, length, or weight) have a unit conversion factor. Unit conversion factors (UCF) may be used in an equation, as shown in Exhibit 3-2, or in a substitution method.

The substitution method is a shortcut that takes the equation directly to the second step of solving for x (Exhibit 3-4). This is possible because UCF equations follow consistent steps and the second step may easily be predicted and used.

How many grams is 4.2 kg?

$$x = 4.2 \text{ kg} \times \frac{1{,}000 \text{ g}}{1 \text{ kg}}$$

$$x = \frac{4.2 \text{ kg}}{1} \times \frac{1{,}000 \text{ g}}{1 \text{ kg}}$$

$$x = \frac{4{,}200 \text{ g}}{1}$$

$$x = 4{,}200 \text{ g}$$

Exhibit 3-4 Substitution Method of Unit Conversion

The key to using this method is to recognize which unit of the UCF must be placed in the numerator. A convenient UCF rule is that the unit asked for in the answer, the "targeted" unit, is placed in the numerator. The starting unit is placed in the denominator.

In setting up unit conversion factor problems, the targeted unit is placed in the numerator, and the starting unit is placed in the denominator.

Exhibit 3-5 Unit Conversion Factor Rule

APOTHECARY MEASUREMENTS

The apothecary system is the measuring system most commonly used in the United States. Length is measured in inches, feet, yards, and miles. Volume is measured in cups, quarts, and gallons. Weight is measured in ounces, pounds, and tons. Scientific applications use metric measures.

Most medications are measured in metric measurements. Occasionally, there may be an apothecary measurement, such as teaspoons or tablespoons, for fluid medication. It may be necessary to make conversions between apothecary and metric units. The most common need is to calculate dosages based on patient weight or to measure size or distance. Most American clinicians think in terms of pounds and feet or inches. It may be necessary to convert these to kilograms and centimeters. The ratios between approximately equal units of measure are listed in Table 3-5.

Table 3-5 Apothecary to Metric Unit Conversion Factors

Apothecary Weight	Metric
2.204 pounds (lb)	1 kilogram (kg)
15.432 grains (gr)	1 gram (g)
Length	
1 inch (in)	2.54 centimeters (cm)
39.37 inches (in)	1 meter (m)
Fluid Volume	
1.057 fluid quart (qt)	1 liter (L)
1 fluid ounce (oz)	28.3 grams (g)

The ratios in Table 3-5 may be used to convert from apothecary to metric or vice versa. The ratios may be manipulated in an equation to suit the clinician's needs. Exhibit 3-6 is a conversion between pounds and kilograms.

HOUSEHOLD MEASUREMENTS

The household measurement system is a system of measuring small volumes of fluid and dry quantities (Exhibit 3-7). It must be stressed that the system is imprecise. Measuring devices such as teaspoons, tablespoons, and

How many kilograms does a 165 lb person weigh?

The most precise unit conversion factor for pounds to kilograms is 2.204 lb:1 kg, but we have rounded the 2.204 lb off to one decimal point and are using 2.2 lb: 1 kg because it is accurate enough.

$$\frac{x}{165 \text{ lb}} = \frac{1 \text{ kg}}{2.2 \text{ lb}}$$

$$\frac{165 \text{ lb } (x)}{165 \text{ lb}} = \frac{(1 \text{ kg}) \ 165 \text{ lb}}{2.2 \text{ lb}}$$

$$x = \frac{165 \text{ kg}}{2.2}$$

$$x = 75 \text{ kg}$$

Exhibit 3-6 Example of Apothecary to Metric Conversion

cups are not precise instruments. The household system is rarely used for prescribing medication. However, **syrups** may be prescribed to be taken by the teaspoon or tablespoon.

1 teaspoon (t)	60 drops 5 milliliters $\frac{1}{8}$ ounce 60 minims 60 grains
1 tablespoon (T)	3 teaspoons $\frac{1}{2}$ fluid ounce 4 drams
1 cup	16 (fluid) tablespoons 12 (dry) tablespoons 8 fluid ounces
1 pint	2 cups 2 glasses 16 ounces $\frac{1}{2}$ quart
Household units of measure are not precise.	

Exhibit 3-7 Household Measures and Weights

A few medications, primarily proteins, are not easily analyzed by laboratory methods. These have measures of medication established by clinical experiments on laboratory animals and subsequently on humans. The measure is called a "unit." There is no precise standard increment of measure for a unit. Insulin is one example of a medication that is measured in units.

Table 3-6 lists the units of measure in each of the three measuring systems. It also displays approximately equal unit ratios of each.

Table 3-6 Comparison of Units of Measure

	Metric	Apothecary	Household*
Weight	64 milligrams	1 grain	none
	1 gram	15.43 grains	none
	1 kilogram	2.204 pounds	none
Volume	1 minim	1 drop	
	1 milliliter	15 minims	15 drops
	3.7 milliliters	1 dram	
	5 milliliters	60 minims	1 teaspoon
	30 milliliters	1 ounce	1 ounce
	1 liter	1.057 quarts	1.057 quarts
Length	1 centimeter	0.3937 inch	none
	2.54 centimeters	1 inch	none
	1 meter	39.37 inches	none

*Household units of measure are not precise.

REVIEW PROBLEMS

Multiply each of the following numbers by the factors shown, and express the answer as a decimal number if it is not a whole number.

	A	B	C
	1,000	0.001	0.01
1. 3.5	_____	_____	_____
2. 35	_____	_____	_____

	A	**B**	**C**
	1,000	0.001	0.01
3. 350	_____	_____	_____
4. 1	_____	_____	_____
5. ¼	_____	_____	_____
6. 50 mg	_____	_____	_____
7. 1,354	_____	_____	_____

Identify the following metric prefixes by the quantity they represent. Include both the fraction expression and the decimal expression.

	Fraction	**Decimal**
Ex. centi	1/100	0.01
8. milli	_____	_____
9. micro	_____	_____
10. nano	_____	_____
11. deka	_____	_____
12. hecto	_____	_____
13. kilo	_____	_____

Identify the following.

14. The metric unit of length is the _____.

15. The metric unit of mass (weight) is the _____.

16. The metric unit of volume is the _____.

17. _____ is the international name for the metric system.

Identify the unit conversion factor for each of the following.

Ex. pounds to kilograms   <u>1 kg/2.2 lb</u>

18. kilograms to pounds   _____

19. grams to kilograms   _____

20. milligrams to grams   _____

21. kilograms to grams   _____

22. grams to milligrams   _____

23. milligrams to nanograms   _____

24. liters to milliliters   _____

25. milliliters to liters   _____

26. milliliters to g (of sterile water)   _____

27. meters to millimeters   _____

28. millimeters to meters   _____

29. meters to centimeters   _____

30. centimeters to meters   _____

31. centimeters to inches   _____

32. inches to centimeters   _____

33. milliliters to ounces   _____

34. ounces to milliliters   _____

35. grams to grains   _____

36. grains to grams   _____

37. milligrams to grains   _____

38. nanograms to milligrams   _____

39. grains to milligrams   _____

40. meters to kilometers   _____

41. kilometers to meters   _____

42. grams to micrograms   _____

43. micrograms to grams   _____

44. milligrams to nanograms   _____

45. nanograms to micrograms   _____

Make the indicated conversions and fill in the following table.

46. 220 lb = _____kg   or   _____mg

47. 0.5 L = _____ml   or   _____dcl (deciliters)

48. 5.0 L = _____ml   or   _____dl (dekaliter)

49. 250 g = _____mg   or   _____ mcg (microgram)

50. 250 mg = _____g   or   _____mcg

51. 250 mcg = _____mg   or   _____ng (nanogram)

52. 250 ml = _____L   or   _____g (of sterile water)

53. 10 gr = _____g   or   _____mg

54. 3 oz = _____ml   or   _____L

55. 60 ml = _____L   or   _____oz

56. 84 kg = _____lb   or   _____mg

57. 220 kg = _____mg   or   _____lb

Arrange the values in Table 3-7 in ascending order.

Table 3-7 Comparisons of Units of Length, Volume, and Weight

Arrange the following from smallest to largest unit of measure:

5 in	5 cm	50 cm	1 yd	1 m
58. ____	59. ____	60. ____	61. ____	62. ____

Arrange the following from smallest to largest unit of measure:

1 qt	1 L	500 ml	5,000 ml	1 gal
63. ____	64. ____	65. ____	66. ____	67. ____

Arrange the following from smallest to largest unit of measure:

49 kg	100 lb	4,900 g	55,000 mg	55,000 g
68. ____	69. ____	70. ____	71. ____	72. ____

Complete the following table of weights.

73. 1 lb = _____kg   or   _____mg

74. 110 lb = _____kg   or   _____mg

75. 184.8 lb = _____kg   or   _____mg

76. 75 kg = _____lb   or   _____mg

77. 466 lb = _____kg   or   _____mg

78. 1 lb = _____g   or   _____gr

79. 1 oz of sterile water = _____g   or   _____mg

80. 1 oz = _____ml   or   _____g (of sterile water)

81. 1 g = _____gr

82. 1 gr = _____mg

83. Explain in what ways the metric system is different from the Arabic number system.

_____

_____

_____

84. Define unit conversion factor.

85. Of the household and metric measuring systems, which is more precise?

_____

_____

_____

Complete the following conversions.

86. 5 L = _____gal

87. 100 ml = _____t

88. 100 ml = _____fluid oz

89. 1 yd = _____m

90. 10 g = _____oz

91. 1 qt = _____L

92. 1 fluid oz = _____ml

93. 1 gal = _____L

94. 1 g = _____gr

95. 1 oz = _____g

96. 1 t = _____ml

97. 1 gr = _____ml

98. 1 ft = _____m

99. 1 in = _____cm

100. 1 yd = _____m

Chapter 4

Mathematical Concepts

> If one is master of one thing and understands one thing well, one has at the same time insight into and understanding of many things.
>
> —Van Gogh.

Exhibit 4-1

Objectives

Upon completion of this chapter the clinician should be able to:

1. Solve basic algebraic equations for x, allowing for precision to the number of significant digits
2. Make necessary metric conversions to solve equations and express the answer with the fewest possible non-integer terms

Key Terms

accuracy	precision
cubic centimeter	quotient
dimension	unit of measure
dimensional unit	word factor

RATIO EQUATIONS WITH METRICS

Word factors are not easily eliminated from an equation. The equation must be factored to create an expression with the same word factor in the numerator and denominator. This creates an expression divided by itself, which is always a **quotient** of 1, thereby dividing out word factors from the expression.

If the original word factor is in the denominator, factoring will require multiplication. If the word factor is in the numerator, factoring will require division. Remember: multiplication and division must be performed equally on both sides of an equation.

Word factors can only be reduced to 1 when they are divided by an exact duplicate of themselves. Therefore, to manipulate **units of measure** in an equation, word factors should be simplified by conversion to like word factors whenever possible.

DIMENSIONS

A **dimension** is a quality of measure. The metric system has three basic dimensions of concern; length, volume, and mass. Within each dimension there are **dimensional units** of measure. For example, in the dimension of mass, the units of measure include gram, milligram, microgram, and kilogram.

All metric expressions of the same dimension (length, volume, or mass) in an equation should be simplified by conversion to like dimensional units (Exhibit 4-2). The use of like units permits factoring the equation to eliminate word factors.

Mass	kilogram	gram	milligram	microgram	nanogram
Volume	liter	milliliter	deciliter	cubic centimeter	
Length	kilometer	meter	centimeter	millimeter	micrometer

Exhibit 4-2 Like Measurements

For example, factors ending in the dimension unit "gram"—such as milligram, microgram, kilogram, or gram—are all units of mass. These should, for medicinal administration, all be converted to the same dimensional unit, such as milligram.

This dimensional conversion rule applies to all metric dimensions used in equations. In the metric dimension of volume, the dimensional units are liter and milliliter. A **cubic centimeter** (cc) is a measurement of area equal to a milliliter. Milliliters and cubic centimeters are frequently used interchangeably. However, when discussing volume (rather than cubic area), milliliter is the most correct expression.

Conversions may be made between units *within* a dimension, such as mass (grams) to mass (milligrams). Conversions cannot be directly made *between* dimensions, such as from mass (grams) to volume (milliliters).

All metric units of the same dimension should be converted to like units.

Conversions cannot be made directly between different dimensions, such as mass (grams) to volume (milliliters).

Exhibit 4-3 Dimensional Conversion Rule

TARGET SELECTION

Once the clinician has decided to simplify an equation with conversions between dimensional units, the target, or unit to which the conversion is to be made, must be selected. For example, does one convert from milligrams to grams or from grams to milligrams? Selecting a target is not critical to the operation. Any dimensional conversion that is mathematically sound will permit solution of the equation. Expressing measurements in a unit that allows the smallest whole number or mixed number (a whole number and a fraction) is helpful when deciding whether to convert to larger or smaller units of measure. Smaller whole numbers are easier to multiply or divide than large numbers. For example, *7.2 kilograms* is easier to work with than 7,200 mg or 7,200,000 mcg. Also as a contrast, 7.2 mg is easier to work with than 0.0072 kg. There are two guiding considerations in selecting the simplest target dimensional unit.

Any dimensional conversion that is mathematically sound will permit solution of an equation.

However, units that allow the clinician to discuss the calculation in integers are preferred.

Exhibit 4-4 Evaluation of the Most Correct Metric Terms

First, in what unit is the medication measured? If possible, all conversions should be made to the unit in which the medication is measured. If a medication is measured in milligrams, the logical target selection is milligrams, and all dimensional units of mass will be converted to milligrams.

Second, which dimensional units will permit the most simplified mathematical operations? If conversion to grams will require arithmetic to the third decimal place, one may wish to work in milligrams to simplify operations.

Exhibit 4-5 is an equation that requires dimensional analysis and conversion of metric word factors. The clinician must convert kilograms and milligrams to a common dimensional unit. In Exhibit 4-5, converting kilograms to milligrams results in a number in the millions.

In the following equation, a conversion must be made to simplify the use of dimensional units.

$$\frac{x}{5 \text{ kg}} = \frac{100 \text{ ml}}{5{,}000 \text{ mg}}$$

Kilograms and milligrams are both units of mass and must be converted to a common dimensional unit to form a common denominator.

Convert kilograms to milligrams.

$$5 \text{ kg} = ? \text{ mg}$$

Conversion from kilograms to milligrams is desired.

$$5 \text{ kg} = \left(\frac{1{,}000{,}000 \text{ mg}}{1 \text{ kg}} \right) = y \text{ mg}$$

The unit conversion factor substitution method is used.

$$5 \text{ kg} = 5{,}000{,}000 \text{ mg}$$

The answer is 5,000,000 mg.

Now the original equation may be expressed:

$$\frac{x}{5{,}000{,}000 \text{ mg}} = \frac{100 \text{ ml}}{5{,}000 \text{ mg}}$$

Substitute 5,000,000 mg for 5 kg in the equation. Now the equation may be solved for x because it has a common denominator.

$$x = 100{,}000 \text{ ml or } 100 \text{ L}$$

Exhibit 4-5 Example Unit Conversion

Conversions that do not simplify the mathematical operation as much as possible still yield correct results. Larger numbers are more difficult to use mathematically. The additional difficulty increases the possibility of error.

A more effective dimensional conversion may be to convert both the kilograms and the milligrams to grams, as in Exhibit 4-6.

Given the following problem, solve for x.

$$\frac{x}{5 \text{ kg}} = \frac{100 \text{ ml}}{5,000 \text{ mg}}$$

Kilograms and milligrams are both units of mass and must be converted to a common dimensional unit and a common denominator.

Convert kilograms and milligrams to grams.

Problem 1: 5 kg = y g
Problem 2: 5,000 mg = z g

Convert from kilograms to grams.
Convert from milligrams to grams.

$$5 \text{ kg} \left(\frac{1,000 \text{ g}}{1 \text{ kg}} \right) = y \text{ g}$$

The unit conversion factor substitution method is used.

5 kg = 5,000 g

The answer is 5,000 g.

A similar operation is used to convert the 5,000 mg to 5 g. Now the original equation may be solved with a common denominator.

$$\frac{x}{5,000 \text{ g}} = \frac{100 \text{ ml}}{5 \text{ g}}$$

Now the equation may be solved for x.

Kilograms and milligrams are both units of mass and must be converted to a common dimensional unit and a common denominator.

$$\frac{x}{5 \text{ kg}} = \frac{100 \text{ ml}}{5,000 \text{ mg}}$$

A similar operation is used to convert the 5,000 mg to 5 g. Now the original equation has units expressed in grams and may be solved using a common denominator.

$$\frac{x}{5,000 \text{ g}} = \frac{100 \text{ ml}}{5 \text{ g}}$$

Now the equation may be solved for x.

$$\cancel{5,000 \text{ g}} \left(\frac{x}{\cancel{5,000 \text{ g}}} \right) = \overset{1,000}{\cancel{5,000 \text{ g}}} \left(\frac{100 \text{ ml}}{\cancel{5 \text{ g}}} \right)$$

x = 100,000 ml

x = 100 L

To reduce a large metric number to a more workable number, we convert milliliters to liters using a unit conversion factor again.

Exhibit 4-6 Example Metric Conversions

Conversions must be made in Exhibit 4-5, Exhibit 4-6, and Exhibit 4-7 to set up a common denominator so the problem can be solved. This will simplify the use of dimensional units.

$$\frac{x}{5\,g} = \frac{1\,ml}{250\,mg}$$

To solve, units in the denominators must be the same denomination. So we can either convert from milligrams to grams or from grams to milligrams. Converting to milligrams will give us whole numbers to work with, while converting to grams will have us working with a decimal number. Either conversion will work, but the author prefers to work with whole numbers, so we will convert to milligrams to give us a common denominator. (The unit conversion operation is not shown in this example.)

$$\frac{x}{5{,}000\,mg} = \frac{1\,ml}{250\,mg}$$

$$\frac{1}{5{,}000\,mg} \left(\frac{x}{5{,}000\,mg} \right)_1 = \left(\frac{1\,ml}{250\,mg} \right)_1 \frac{20}{5{,}000\,mg}$$

$x = 20\ ml$

Exhibit 4-7 Example Metric Conversion with Unit Conversion Factor Substitution

60 min/hr
100¢/4 quarters
100¢/$1
52 weeks/year
4 quarters/$1
2.2 lb/kg
12/1 dozen
1,000 ml/L
16 oz/1 lb

Exhibit 4-8 Example Unit Conversion Factors

ACCURACY

Scientists, including health care professionals, make a distinction between **accuracy** and precision. Accuracy is to be free from error, but not necessarily exact. It refers to how closely a measured or estimated value agrees with the correct value. An approximation may be accurate. Patients rarely appreciate having their medication doses approximated.

PRECISION

Precision is accurate, correct, and as exact as possible. The amount of exactness is determined by the exactness of the other numbers used in the mathematical operation. For example, if an order for medication reads "give 1 mg per kilogram," the closest precision is a whole kilogram of patient weight, or in the case of a neonate or a premature infant, the order may even be given per unit of body weight in grams. Doses for neonates must be very precise. It is not possible to be more precise than the numbers in the initial problem. A tenth of a kilogram or one hundredth of a kilogram in this problem is not significant.

SIGNIFICANT DIGITS

Some digits are exact (or precise) numbers that are known to be absolutely accurate. These include scientific constants, such as the speed of light. Other numbers are accurate and only precise to the number of significant digits. The measurements on medication labels are exact.

Significant digits are numbers obtained by measurement and believed to be correct by the clinician making the measurement. The patient's weight is a number limited by the precision of the instrument used to weigh the patient. For example, a scale that measures in whole kilograms cannot be used to determine weight more precisely than a whole kilogram. It cannot precisely determine the weight to hundredths of a kilogram.

Any mathematical operation can only be as precise as the least precise factor in it.

Exhibit 4-9 Rule of Significant Digits

Rules of significant digits:

1. Leading or trailing zeros that hold decimal places are not significant digits. For example, 0.025 has only two significant digits. Also 0.205 has 3 significant digits because the middle zero is neither a leading or trailing zero.
2. In multiplication and division, a precise answer can have significant digits no more precise than the factor with least number of significant digits used in the operation.
3. In addition and subtraction, the last digit retained in the answer is determined by the least precise digit.

For an example equation using significant numbers, see Exhibit 4-10.

Consider the equation 1.2 * 3.111113. It will give an answer significant only to the one decimal point because 1.2 is the limiting number of significant digits, and it has two significant digits. The other number, 3.111113, has seven significant figures, but the answer can only be as significant as the least precise number used in deriving it.

1.2 * 3.111113 = 3.7333356

The answer will, for scientific and medical use, be rounded off to 3.7. Only one decimal point is significant because the least precise number in the problem was 1.2 and it has one place after the decimal point.

Exhibit 4-10 Significant Digits in Calculations

Rounding Off

The number of significant digits determines the number of decimal places to which the problem can be precisely calculated. A problem is calculated to one more decimal place than the number of significant digits and then rounded off.

Rounding off is performed by evaluating the last decimal place. If it is five or greater, the preceding decimal place is rounded up to the next digit. If it is less than five, the preceding decimal place is left as it is. The last decimal place is then dropped from the number, as shown in Exhibit 4-11.

3.246	is rounded to	3.25
3.244	is rounded to	3.24
4.26	is rounded to	4.3
4.24	is rounded to	4.2
3.54	is rounded to	3.5

Exhibit 4-11 Rounding Off

Most Appropriate Expression

Metric expressions may be interchanged without loss of precision. For example: 1,500 mg and 1.5 g are the same quantity. (Note: 1,505 mg is more precise than 1,500 mg.) These two expressions are equally correct and precise. However, one is more appropriate than the other. The most appropriate expression is 1.5 g.

Two considerations guide the clinician in determining which expression is the most appropriate:

1. The expression with the lowest whole numbers is appropriate. For example, 5 g is more appropriate than 5,000 mg or 5,000,000 mcg.
2. The solution to an expression cannot be more precise than the initial number of significant digits.

REVIEW PROBLEMS

Solve the following equations for *x*. Make any necessary dimensional conversions.

1. $\dfrac{4x}{2\,L} = \dfrac{4\,mg}{2\,ml}$

2. $\dfrac{4x}{2\,mg} = \dfrac{4\,ml}{2\,g}$

3. $\dfrac{x}{1\,L} = \dfrac{1\,mg}{1\,ml}$

4. $\dfrac{x}{1\,ml} = \dfrac{1\,g}{2\,L}$

5. $\dfrac{x}{110\,lb} = \dfrac{1\,mg}{1\,kg}$

6. $\dfrac{x}{1\,kg} = \dfrac{10\,mg}{1\,lb}$

7. $\dfrac{x}{50\,mg} = \dfrac{110\,lb}{1\,kg}$

8. $\dfrac{x}{10\,mg} = \dfrac{1\,kg}{1\,lb}$

9. $\dfrac{x}{1\,mg} = \dfrac{1\,ml}{1\,L}$

10. $\dfrac{x}{1\,g} = \dfrac{1\,ml}{2\,L}$

11. $\dfrac{x}{50\,mg} = \dfrac{5\,ml}{1\,g}$

12. $\dfrac{x}{50\,mg} = \dfrac{1\,ml}{50\,mcg}$

13. $\dfrac{x}{5\,ml} = \dfrac{50\,mg}{1\,g}$

14. $\dfrac{x}{1\,ml} = \dfrac{50\,mg}{50\,mcg}$

15. $\dfrac{x}{5\,g} = \dfrac{5\,ml}{250\,g}$

16. $\dfrac{x}{1\,g} = \dfrac{1\,tablet}{250\,mg}$

17. $\dfrac{x}{5\,ml} = \dfrac{5\,g}{250\,mg}$

18. $\dfrac{x}{1\,tablet} = \dfrac{1\,g}{250\,mg}$

19. $\dfrac{x}{0.5\,mg} = \dfrac{1\,ml}{1\,mg}$

20. $\dfrac{x}{500\,mg} = \dfrac{10\,ml}{1\,g}$

21. $\dfrac{x}{1\,ml} = \dfrac{0.5\,mg}{1\,mg}$

22. $\dfrac{x}{10\,ml} = \dfrac{500\,mg}{1\,g}$

23. $\dfrac{x}{30\ \text{ml}} = \dfrac{60\ \text{gtt}}{1\ \text{ml}}$

24. $\dfrac{x}{1\ \text{min}} = \dfrac{120\ \text{ml}}{1\ \text{hr}}$

25. $\dfrac{x}{60\ \text{gtt}} = \dfrac{30\ \text{ml}}{1\ \text{ml}}$

26. $\dfrac{x}{120\ \text{ml}} = \dfrac{1\ \text{min}}{1\ \text{hr}}$

27. $\dfrac{x}{90\%} = \dfrac{10\ \text{ml}}{100\%}$

28. $\dfrac{x}{33.3\%} = \dfrac{333\ \text{mg}}{100\%}$

29. $\dfrac{x}{10\ \text{ml}} = \dfrac{90\%}{100\%}$

30. $\dfrac{x}{333\ \text{mg}} = \dfrac{33.3\%}{100\%}$

31. $\dfrac{x}{15\ \text{mg}} = \dfrac{1\ \text{ml}}{1\ \text{mg}}$

32. $\dfrac{x}{180\ \text{ml}} = \dfrac{10\ \text{gtt}}{1\ \text{ml}}$

33. $\dfrac{x}{1\ \text{ml}} = \dfrac{15\ \text{mg}}{1\ \text{mg}}$

34. $\dfrac{x}{110\ \text{lb}} = \dfrac{1\ \text{ml}}{8\ \text{oz}}$

35. $\dfrac{x}{1\ \text{min}} = \dfrac{60\ \text{ml}}{1\ \text{hr}}$

36. $\dfrac{x}{1\ \text{min}} = \dfrac{1{,}440\ \text{ml}}{1\ \text{day}}$

37. $\dfrac{x}{5\ \text{ml}} = \dfrac{40\ \text{mg}}{1\ \text{L}}$

38. $\dfrac{x}{5\ \text{min}} = \dfrac{4\ \text{mg}}{1\ \text{hr}\ 40\ \text{min}}$

39. $\dfrac{x}{0.005\ \text{L}} = \dfrac{0.04\ \text{g}}{1\ \text{L}}$

40. $\dfrac{x}{24\ \text{hr}} = \dfrac{2\ \text{tablets}}{4\ \text{hr}}$

Identify the number of significant digits in the expressions below.

41. 0.0002 _____   42. 0.1002 _____

43. 5,000 mg _____   44. 5,001 g _____

45. 2 mg _____   46. 40 kg _____

47. 0.5 mg _____

Which of the following units are units of the same dimension?

48. _____   and   _____

millimeters
cubic grams
cubic centimeters
centimeters

49. _____ and _____

grams
milliliters
kilometers
micrograms

50. _____ and _____

meters
milligrams
kiloliters
centimeters

Chapter 5

Word Problems

"Then you should say what you mean," the March Hare went on.

"I do," Alice hastily replied, "at least—at least I mean what I say—that's the same thing, you know."

"Not the same thing a bit!" said the Hatter. "Why you might just as well say that 'I see what I eat' is the same thing as 'I eat what I see'!"

—Lewis Carroll, *Alice's Adventures in Wonderland.*

Exhibit 5-1

OBJECTIVES

Upon completion of this chapter the clinician should be able to:

1. List three steps in setting up equations to solve dosage calculation problems from verbal orders

2. Set up word problems as algebraic equations

3. Solve algebraic equations, making necessary unit conversions to express the answer with the fewest non-integer factors

4. Given a concentration for a medicine, calculate the mass for any volume

5. Given a concentration for a medicine, calculate the volume for any mass

KEY TERMS

bolus

concentration

infusion

mass

mEq

milliequivalent

order of operations

sum

volume

WORD PROBLEMS

Physician orders for medication are often given verbally. This extends the physician's responsibility to the clinician. The clinician is ethically and legally responsible to administer the correct amount of medication. No health care provider should administer any medications or dose unless he is absolutely certain it is correct.

No health care provider should administer any dose until absolutely certain it is correct.

Exhibit 5-2 Clinician Responsibility

A clinician who is uncertain about a medication should advise the physician, check reference sources, and question the order. The clinician must confirm the following eight things: (1) the medication is right; (2) the dose is right; (3) the route is right; (4) the time for the dose is right; (5) it is being given to the right patient (confirm a written identification); (6) the patient has no medication allergies; (7) the patient consents to treatment; and (8) the clinician properly documents the medication administration. If the clinician's concern about any one of these is not resolved, he should advise the physician that he is unable to carry out the order and ask for an alternative. Some physicians may feel this challenges their authority, but most will appreciate the clinician's professionalism. Court cases have established the precedent that the clinician is personally responsible for medications he administers, even if complying with a physician's incorrect order.

Approach to Word Problems

The correct dose for some verbal orders is easily deduced intuitively, in the clinician's thoughts, without setting up an equation. This shortcut has risks. There is an increased risk of error when the clinician does not understand the process by which the answer is derived. Intuitive deduction can cause the clinician difficulty when he encounters more challenging problems. Without practice at setting up necessary equations, a clinician may be unable to solve the problem.

Setting up equations is simple if an organized process is used. There are three basic steps common to setting up an equation to solve any dosage calculation word problem:

1. Identify what is known. This includes what is spoken in an order. It also includes information available on the medication container. The

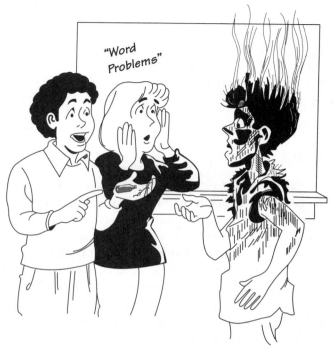

"No, no! I said nitroglycerine **PILLS**"

Figure 5-1 Nitroglycerine

medication container gives a concentration ratio of mass (usually grams or milliliters) to milliliters (or liters). Known information also includes basic knowledge, such as a working familiarity of the metric system.

2. Identify what is unknown and is asked for. A problem may have preliminary steps before the measured dose may be calculated (such as converting units of measure to like units). Many students have difficulty interpreting word problems, but once the *needed* information is identified, a ratio equation, using the known information, can be set up to solve for the unknown data. The clinician usually must know the metric dose or volume of the dose. One of those is usually given, and the other must be calculated.

3. Set up a ratio equation to solve for the unknown information. Many equations require a known concentration ratio. They also require either the volume or the weight of medication. An equation can only be solved for one unknown. Problems that require a solution for more than one unknown factor must have an equation for each.

---

1. Identify what is known.

2. Identify what is unknown.

3. Set up an equation and solve for the unknown.

Exhibit 5-3 Three Steps to Solving Word Problems

CONCENTRATIONS

There are several types of problems associated with verbal orders. These include calculation of infusion drip rates, mixing new concentrations, amount of medicine per unit of patient body weight, and rate of administration. The most common is concentration analysis.

Most verbal medication orders require calculating a volume of medication based on a mass. These are concentration problems. **Concentration** may be defined as an unchanging ratio of units of mass to units of volume.

Mass may be defined in this context as the weight of medicine. This is a bit simplified. The full scientific definition includes other considerations not necessary for dosage calculation.

Volume is the space occupied by a body. Most medications are fluid. A fluid volume of medication is most correctly expressed in dimensions of liters, such as milliliters (ml) or liters (L), rather than cubic area such as centimeters (cc).

In concentration problems, the concentration is provided on the medication label. A constant relationship exists between the units of volume and mass. The concentration may be used to determine any unit of mass for any given related unit of volume. Likewise, it may be used to determine any unit of volume for any given related unit of mass.

A concentration may be used to determine any unit of mass for any related unit of volume or any unit of volume for any related unit of mass.

Exhibit 5-4 Concentration

The form in which the concentration is used in an equation is not limited by how it is expressed. It may be used with either part (mass or volume) of the expression in the numerator.

   The manner in which a concentration is set up in an equation is determined by the unknown. The easiest manner to set up an equation is to
place the unknown in the numerator. Place the related known concentration (or volume) in the denominator. The given concentration is then set
up on the other side of the equation in a parallel manner (if volume is on
the bottom, the denominator) on the left, place volume on the bottom on
the right), as shown in Exhibit 5-5. If x, the unknown, has milligrams in the
denominator, then the concentration will be set up with milligrams in the
denominator. If x has milliliters in the denominator, then the concentration
will have milliliters in the denominator. See Exhibit 5-6 and Exhibit 5-7
for example concentration problems.

The unknown is set up in the numerator as x, and its related reference is placed in
the denominator. The concentration is then set up in a parallel form.

$$\frac{x}{\text{ordered volume}} = \frac{\text{given mass}}{\text{given volume}}$$

There is parallelism between the denominators and numerators.

Exhibit 5-5 Setting Up Concentration Problems

Given a concentration of 100 mg/10 ml:

The physician order is to give 5 ml. How many milligrams are given?

First: The concentration is known to be 100 mg/10 ml.
                The dose volume is known to be 5 ml.

Second: The unknown element is the metric dose.

Third: To set up the equation, we begin with the left side of the equation
                as x and then plug in the known data. We will place the metric dose
                of the concentration in the numerator because the metric dose of
                the order is what we are seeking.

$$\frac{x}{5 \text{ ml}} = \frac{100 \text{ mg}}{10 \text{ ml}}$$

The last step is to solve for x, which is 50 mg.

Exhibit 5-6 Example Concentration Problem

The same problem in Exhibit 5-6 could be set up to ask for the dose volume instead of the metric dose. We merely set up the equation with volume in the numerator.

Given a concentration of 100 mg/10 ml:

The physician order is to give 50 mg. How many milliliters are given?

First: The concentration is known to be 100 mg/10 ml.
 The metric dose is known to be 50 mg.

Second: The unknown element is the dose volume.

Third: To set up the equation, we begin with the left side of the equation as x and then plug in the known data. We will place the volume of the concentration in the numerator because the dose volume of the order is what we are seeking.

$$\frac{x}{50 \text{ mg}} = \frac{10 \text{ ml}}{100 \text{ mg}}$$

The last step is to solve for x, which is 5 ml.

Exhibit 5-7 Example Concentration Problem

A three-part concentration such as:

factor:	100 mg /	10 ml /	prefilled syringe
	—	—	—
part:	1	2	3

will have only two of the three parts used at one time. Any two of the three may be used in a parallel set-up. Exhibit 5-8 solves first for the metric dose, as Exhibit 5-7 did, and then solves for the number of syringes. The point of this example is that any part of a concentration can be used to solve a question.

A solution measured in percent (%) indicates a ratio of medication per 100 ml of solution. Calcium chloride is an electrolyte. Electrolytes are measured in milliequivalents rather than grams or milliliters and is expressed in percent.

Presupplied electrolyte solutions can be another example of a multiple-part ratio. A medication is supplied in prefilled syringes of a 10% solution containing 1 g of medication in 10 ml. Electrolytic solutions are measured

Given a concentration of 100 mg/10 ml/prefilled syringe:

The physician order is for 5 ml. How many milligrams are given?

First: The concentration is known to be 100 mg/10 ml/1 syringe.

Second: We are asked for the metric dose in milligrams.
Third: We set up an equation and place the metric dose
                in the numerator.

$$\frac{x}{} = \frac{}{}$$ Start with our standard equation form.

$$\frac{x}{5\ ml} = \frac{100\ mg}{10\ ml}$$ We plug in the known data and
                solve for x, which is 50 mg.

The clinician needs to know how many prefilled syringes will be needed to give the dose. An equation can be used to find the number of syringes.

The same three steps are used. The second step now asks for syringes instead of the metric dose.

$$x = \frac{}{}$$ Start with our standard equation form.

$$\frac{x}{50\ mg} = \frac{1\ syringe}{100\ mg}$$ We plug in the known data and
                solve for x, which is 0.5 syringes.

Exhibit 5-8 Example Concentration Problem

in **milliequivalents (mEq)**. There are 13.6 mEq in a 10 ml syringe of 10% solution. The supply ratio for this medication has four parts, as shown in Exhibit 5-9. See Exhibit 5-10 for a sample problem using milliequivalents. Many electrolyte solutions are too concentrated for administration to infants, children, or patients with compromised circulation. A clinician must be prepared to dilute a premixed solution to a lower concentration to safely administer it.

Concentration	1 prefilled syringe/	1 g/	10 ml/	13.6 mEq
Part	1	2	3	4

Exhibit 5-9 Electrolyte Concentration

You are supplied a prefilled syringe with 1 g of an electrolytic medication in a 10 ml syringe of 10% solution containing 13.6 mEq (milliequivalents).

The physician orders you to give 20 mEq. How many milliliters do you administer, and how many prefilled syringes will you need to give it?

First: Known data: 1 g/   10 ml/   10%/   13.6 mEq/   1 syringe
        Physician's order: 20 mEq
        This is a lot of data, so we need to organize it to see what we
        need to solve the problem and leave out what we don't need.

Second: Needed data: ? ml   ? mEq

Third: $\dfrac{x}{} = \underline{}$ Start with our standard equation.

$\dfrac{x}{20 \text{ mEq}} = \dfrac{10 \text{ ml}}{13.6 \text{ mEq}}$ Plug in the known data.
Solve for x.

$(\cancel{20 \text{ mEq}}) \dfrac{x}{\cancel{20 \text{ mEq}}} = \dfrac{10 \text{ ml}}{13.6 \cancel{\text{ mEq}}} (20 \cancel{\text{ mEq}})$

$x = \dfrac{200 \text{ ml}}{13.6}$ Solve for x.

$x = 14.7$ ml   This gives us the volume of the dose.

To solve for the number of syringes, we use the same first and second steps and set up the equation for syringes instead of milliequivalents.

$\dfrac{x}{20 \text{ mEq}} = \dfrac{1 \text{ syringe}}{13.6 \text{ mEq}}$

$x = 1.47$ syringes. The problem has only two significant figures, so the answer is rounded to 1.5 syringes, which is two significant figures.

Common sense tells us syringes are counted in whole numbers, so while we only give medication of 1.5 syringes, we will need 2 syringes, which is the closest whole number above 1.5.

Exhibit 5-10 Example Milliequivalent Problem

Any two parts of this "supply ratio" may be used in a parallel manner in an equation.

See Exhibit 5-11: an order is given for 75 mg of 2% lidocaine to be given as an IV bolus. The syringe is measured in milliliters, not milligrams.

The physician orders 75 mg of 2% lidocaine to be administered. The medication is packaged in a syringe of 100 mg/5 ml.

First: The concentration is known to be   100 mg/5 ml.
                 The metric dose is known to be   75 mg.

Second: The unknown element is the dose volume in milliliters.

Third: Set up an equation.

$$\frac{x}{\rule{2cm}{0.4pt}} = \frac{}{\rule{2cm}{0.4pt}}$$

$$\frac{x}{75 \text{ mg}} = \frac{5 \text{ ml}}{100 \text{ mg}}$$ Milliliters are needed, so we set up the concentration side of the equation with milliliters in the numerator.

$$(\cancel{75 \text{ mg}}) \; \frac{x}{\cancel{75 \text{ mg}}} = \frac{5 \text{ ml}}{100 \text{ mg}} \; (\cancel{75 \text{ mg}})$$

$$x = \frac{375 \text{ ml}}{100}$$

$$x = 3.75 \text{ ml}$$

Exhibit 5-11 Example Concentration Problem

How much medication (in milliliters) is used from the syringe to give 75 mg?

See Exhibit 5-12. A physician orders medication in a dose of 5 mg/kg of patient weight to be given as an IV bolus. The medication is supplied in a pre-filled syringe measured in milliliters. How much medication is used from the syringe to give 5 mg/kg? The patient weighs 132 lb. The medication label reads "500 mg/10 ml" in the prefilled syringe.

Exhibit 5-12 is a concentration problem. Given an order for medication based on patient weight, the clinician must calculate both the mass and the related volume for the dose. Solution of this problem requires more than one step because the related mass is not *directly* given. The related mass is expressed in milligrams per kilogram of patient weight. Patient weight is expressed in pounds.

There are three problems to be solved: first, the patient's weight in kilograms; second, the related mass of medicine; and third, the related volume of the medicine to be given. The number of calculations adds complexity to the question, but a step-by-step approach using the equation set-up process simplifies it. Each calculation gives additional data used for the next step.

This problem involves three calculations. The order is based on patient weight in kilograms. The first calculation will be the patient's weight in kilograms. The second calculation will be the metric dose, and the third will be the dose volume. We can use x, y, and z for the unknown to distinguish between each of the calculations.

First: Concentration: 500 mg/10 ml
               Order: 5 mg/kg patient weight
               Patient weight: 132 lb
               Unit conversion factor for kilograms: 2.204 lb/1 kg

Second: Needed: patient weight in kilograms
                              metric dose in milligrams
                              dose volume in milliliters

Third: $\dfrac{x}{}$ = $\underline{}$

$\dfrac{x}{132\text{ lb}} = \dfrac{1\text{ kg}}{2.2\text{ lb}}$

We set up a unit conversion factor to calculate patient weight. There are only two significant figures to this, so we can use 2.2 with adequate accuracy.

$x = 60$ kg

This is the patient weight in kilograms.

$\dfrac{y}{60\text{ kg}} = \dfrac{5\text{ mg}}{1\text{ kg}}$

We set up the second calculation, which is for the metric dose. Milligrams are in the numerator because that is what is needed.

$y = 300$ mg

This is the metric dose.

$\dfrac{z}{300\text{ mg}} = \dfrac{10\text{ ml}}{500\text{ mg}}$

We set up the third calculation, which is for dose volume. Milliliters are in the numerator because that is what is needed.

$z = 6$ ml

This is the dose volume.

Exhibit 5-12 Example Concentration Problem

INFUSION AND BOLUS

Some of the terms used in verbal orders specify the manner in which a medication is to be administered. Intravenous therapy may be either by infusion or by bolus.

Infusion is a prolonged, controlled introduction of fluid into the body. This allows a very controlled rate of medication administration. Rates of infusion administration are commonly calculated in milliliters per hour. Intravenous (IV) infusions allow medications that may be too caustic or too concentrated for normal IV injection to be given intravenously in a diluted mixture. Infusion calculations are discussed in Chapter 8.

A mass of medication given as a single unit is a **bolus**. An IV bolus is a unit of medication injected as a single dose into a vein. The rate of the bolus injection depends on the medication being given. Intravenous boluses of small amounts should usually be given over 5 to 10 minutes. This provides the medication at a rate best suited to the body's ability to adsorb it. A rare number of medications must be given by rapid IV bolus (as quickly as possible) but most are administered during 5 to 10 minutes. A clinician must know the recommended routes and rates of each medication before administering it. It is usually the route of choice for administering medication in emergencies.

Total Daily Dose

A total daily dosage is the **sum** of all individual doses given in a 24-hour day. Occasionally, it may be necessary to determine an individual dose based on the total daily dosage and the number of times during the day the medication is given. Frequently used abbreviations to indicate the number of doses in a day include BID for twice a day, TID for three times a day, and QID for four times a day. A list of additional abbreviations is included in Appendix B.

Order of Operations

Mathematical **order of operations** refers to the sequence in which multiple mathematical operations should be performed if there is more than one type of operation in an equation. This was discussed in Chapter 2. A clinician should use parentheses to indicate the order of operations in equations that involve complex mathematical operations.

REVIEW PROBLEMS

Given the concentration on the left, calculate the metric dose for the concentration per unit of volume.

1. 1 g/L _____ mg/ml _____ mg/500 ml

2. 2 g/L _____ mg/ml _____ g/500 ml

3. 1 mg/L _____ mcg/ml _____ mg/500 ml

4. 1 mcg/L _____ ng/ml _____ mcg/250 ml

5. 1 mg/0.5 L _____ mcg/ml _____ mcg/250 ml

6. 1 mg/0.25 L _____ mg/L _____ mcg/ml

7. 2 g/0.5 L   _____ g/250 ml   _____ mg/ml

8. 4 mg/ml   _____ g/L   _____ g/250 ml

9. 4 mcg/ml   _____ mg/L   _____ mg/250 ml

10. 4 mcg/ml   _____ mcg/250 ml   _____ mcg/L

Solve the following word problems using the partial equation provided. The unknown and its related factor are set up. Identify the proper ratio to use, complete the equation, and solve for *x*. Remember to use parallelism in the set-up.

11. How many grams would a clinician administer if a physician ordered 5 mg of morphine sulphate? It is supplied in a 15 mg/ml vial. _____

12. A physician ordered 0.10 g of lidocaine. How many milligrams will the clinician administer? It is supplied in 100 mg/10 ml prefilled syringe. _____

13. How many milliliters are in 0.25 L? _____

14. If a physician ordered 2.5 L of dextrose 5% in water, how many milliliters should be given? _____

15. The order is to give 2 tablets of acetylsalicylic acid. The tablets contain 350 mg of medication each. What is the metric dose given (in milligrams)? _____

16. A physician orders a bolus of lidocaine based on the ratio of 1 mg/kg of patient body weight. The patient weighs 110 lb. The lidocaine is supplied in 100 mg/10 ml syringe. How many milligrams does the clinician administer? _____

17. The label of a vial of medication reads "100 mg/10 ml." If the clinician is giving 1 mg/kg for a 110 lb patient, how many milliliters are administered? _____

18. The order is to give 50 mg. The label of the medication reads "1 g/10 ml." How many milliliters does the clinician administer? _____

19. One dose of a medication is 1 g. It is given TID. How many grams are given in a day? _____

20. A total day's dosage is 4 g. It is administered QID. How much medication is given with each dose? _____

21. A physician orders 10 mg/lb (of patient body weight). The patient weighs 45.45 kg. What is the dose? _____

22. A physician orders 5 mg of morphine sulphate, given BID. What is the total daily dose? _____

23. A physician orders 75 mg of meperidine for a patient. It is supplied in a 50 mg/ml vial. The vial contains 15 ml. How many milliliters does the clinician administer? _____

24. The doctor's orders read: "give 160 mg furosemide." It comes supplied in a container labeled "40 mg/ml." How many milliliters does the clinician administer? _____

25. If 8 ml contains 100 mg, how many milliliters contain 1,250 mg? _____

Use the following information to answer problems 26–28.

A 45.45 kg patient is prescribed 10 mg/lb of a medication to be given TID. The medication is marked "1 g/10 ml."

26. What is the dose? _____
27. How many milliliters are administered? _____
28. What is the total daily dose? _____

Solve problems 29–30 using the following information. Identify the proper ratio to use, set up an equation, and solve for *x*.

The doctor's order is for 1 mg of lidocaine per kilogram of patient body weight. The patient weighs 275 lb. The lidocaine is marked "2% solution, 100 mg/5 ml."

29. How many milligrams does the clinician administer? _____
30. How many milliliters does the clinician administer? _____

Solve problem 31 using the following information. Identify the proper ratio to use, set up an equation, and solve for *x*.

An order is given for 0.5 mg of atropine. It is supplied in a vial marked "1 g/30 ml."

31. How many milliliters does the clinician administer? _____

Solve problems 32–33 using the following information. Identify the proper ratio to use, set up an equation, and solve for *x*.

The doctor in question 31 decided to have the clinician use prefilled syringes, which contain 0.4 mg atropine each. Each syringe is 2 ml in volume.

32. How many prefilled syringes will the clinician use? _____
33. How many milliliters will the clinician administer? _____

Solve problems 34–35 using the following information. Identify the proper ratio to use, set up an equation, and solve for *x*.

A physician orders one half of a 10 ml prefilled syringe of calcium chloride to be administered. The prefilled syringe contains 1 g of 10% medication.

34. How much medication does the clinician administer? _____
35. How many milliliters does the clinician administer? _____

Solve problems 36–38 using the following information. Identify the proper ratio to use, set up an equation, and solve for x.

The doctor's orders are to administer 500 mg of a medication per mouth QID. The medication is supplied in 125 mg units.

36. How many units are given in each dose? ———
37. How many doses are given in a 24-hour day? ———
38. How many total units are given in a day? ———

Solve problems 39–40 using the following information. Identify the proper ratio to use, set up an equation, and solve for x.

A paramedic received an order to administer 1.5 mg/lb of patient body weight to a patient who weighs 90.9 kg. The medication is supplied in a vial containing 1 g in 10 ml.

39. How many milligrams does the clinician administer? ———
40. How many milliliters does the clinician administer? ———

Solve problems 41–43 using the following information. Identify the proper ratio to use, set up an equation, and solve for x.

A physician orders 20 ml of calcium chloride. Calcium chloride is supplied in prefilled syringes of 10% solution containing 10 ml and 1 g and 13.6 mEq.

41. How many milligrams does the patient receive? ———
42. How many syringes are used? ———
43. How many milliequivalents are given? ———

Solve problems 44–45 using the following information. Identify the proper ratio to use, set up an equation, and solve for x.

A patient weighs 185 lb. A physician orders a bolus of lidocaine based on the ratio of 1 mg/kg of body weight for this patient. The medication is supplied in a prefilled syringe of 100 mg/10 ml.

44. How many milligrams are given? ———
45. How many milliliters are given? ———

46. Define parallelism and how it applies to setting up dosage calculation equations.

_____

_____

_____

47. Define concentration.

_____

_____

_____

List the three steps to setting up an equation.

48. _____

49. _____

50. _____

Special Problems

Exhibit 6-1

OBJECTIVES

Upon completion of this chapter the clinician should be able to:

1. Discuss mixing a powdered medication for injection
2. Make decimal conversions
3. Convert Arabic numbers to percent numbers
4. Identify absolute values of positive and negative numbers
5. Determine time on a 24-hour clock

KEY TERMS

absolute value
decimal
negative
percent

plunger
positive
reconstitution

RECONSTITUTION OF POWDERS

Some medications are supplied in a sealed vial as a powder. Many medications have a short shelf life when in solution and are stored in powder form to keep them active. Other medications may be supplied in powder form to permit a wide variety of concentrations.

Medications supplied in powder form must be reconstituted before being injected. **Reconstitution** is the process of mixing the powder with sterile water, saline, or some other solvent to form a solution.

The clinician may encounter difficulty in mixing a powder with a solvent to get a specific concentration, such as 100 mg in 5 ml. The clinician cannot simply add 5 ml of sterile water to 100 mg of powder. The powder itself takes up physical space. If 5 ml of water is added, the mixture will have a total volume greater than 5 ml because of the displacement by the powder (Exhibit 6-2).

The manufacturer may include on the label instructions on how much solvent (fluid) to add to the vial. This simplifies the operation. Any special requirements for storage or reconstitution will also be listed on the label.

Powder cannot be drawn into a syringe, so the powder must be mixed into solution while in its own vial. First, determine how many milliliters of solution are desired. Then, using a syringe, draw that amount of air out of the vial. If the vial is airtight, you will have difficulty injecting the solution if you do not first evacuate the same amount of air. Second, draw up into the syringe a smaller amount of solvent than is desired. Use this syringe to slowly add to the vial just enough solvent to completely dissolve the medication. If the powder does not dissolve easily, gently agitate the vial by moving it in a circular motion as the solvent is added. After the powder dissolves, draw the mixture into a graduated syringe. Then draw up additional solvent, adding to the mixture until the desired number of milliliters for the solution is reached in the syringe.

A clinician may encounter a problem when the physician orders less than the entire amount of medication in the vial. The problem at this point becomes a concentration problem, as discussed in Chapter 5. For example, the vial contains 1,000 mg (or 1 g) of powdered medication. The doctor's order calls for 100 mg. The full amount of powder must be reconstituted, the volume measured, and the concentration determined. The dose is then calculated from the concentration (milligrams per milliliters) of the solution. The balance of medication may be wasted (intentionally discarded) or saved for additional doses. Label the syringe with the medication, the concentration, the metric dose, and your name.

The physician's order may also be to administer a specific concentration of medication. The concentration may be used, with the related mass of medication (from the medication label), to determine the volume of the final solution.

A vial contains 1 g of powdered medication. The doctor orders 100 mg given in a 5 ml bolus.

First: Concentration is 100 mg/5 ml.
Metric dose is 100 mg.
Total metric med is 1 g.

Second: The total amount of solvent (in milliliters) to add to 1 g is needed.

Third: $\dfrac{x}{} = \dfrac{}{}$

$\dfrac{x}{1g} = \dfrac{5 \text{ ml}}{100 \text{ mg}}$ Set up the equation with milliliters in the numerator because that is what we need to calculate.

$\dfrac{x}{1{,}000 \text{ mg}} = \dfrac{5 \text{ ml}}{100 \text{ mg}}$ Convert 1 g to 1,000 mg using the unit conversion factor substitution.

$x = 50 \text{ ml}$ Solve for x.

x is the total amount of solution (including the volume of the powder), so a clinician cannot simply add 50 ml of solvent. The volume of solvent must be less than 50 ml. Add solvent to the powder until there is a total (of solvent and medication) of 50 ml to mix the solution. A clinician could start with about 30 ml of solvent to create the solution and then, after the powder is dissolved, add solvent to a total of 50 ml.

Exhibit 6-2 Calculating Reconstitution Volume

PERCENT

Percent is a portion of the whole divided by 100. It is represented by the symbol %.

A percent is represented by the symbol %. To convert from a percent to a decimal fraction, divide the percent by 100%.

Exhibit 6-3 Converting a Percent to a Decimal Fraction

Conversion of a percent to a **decimal** form is performed by dividing the percent by 100%, as shown in Exhibit 6-4. Division by 100 is sometimes described as moving the decimal two places to the left. The percent symbol is a word factor that must be manipulated mathematically like other word factors. The percent sign is divided by itself and factors out.

To convert 50% to a decimal number, divide the percent by 100%.

$$x = \frac{50\%}{100\%}$$

$$x = \frac{5\cancel{0}\%}{10\cancel{0}\%}$$

$$x = 0.5$$

Exhibit 6-4 Example Conversion of a Percent to a Decimal Fraction

Conversion of any number to a percent is performed by multiplying the number by 100%, as shown in Exhibit 6-5. Multiplying by 100 is sometimes described as moving the decimal two places to the right.

To convert 0.50 to a percent, multiply the number by 100%.

$$x = 0.50 * 100\%$$

$$x = 50\%$$

Exhibit 6-5 Example Conversion of a Decimal Number to a Percent

ABSOLUTE VALUE

Absolute value refers to quantity. Mathematical operations follow precise rules that may yield results with a **negative** sign. To calculate a quantity in a hole 1 ft (foot) wide, 1 ft long, and 1 ft deep would yield an answer of –1 cubic ft.

The great English author Lewis Carroll wrote in *Alice's Adventures in Wonderland*:

> "Take some more tea," the March Hare said to Alice, very earnestly. "I've had nothing yet," Alice replied in an offended tone. "So I can't take more." "You mean you can't take less," said the Hatter. "It's very easy to take more than nothing."[1]

In the measurement of absolute value, you can actually have a **positive** value that represents less than nothing. For example, the Hatter could have given Alice a cup of tea to replace what she did not have. A contractor who wants to purchase concrete to fill the hole will use an "absolute," or real,

---

[1] Carroll, L. (1898). *Alice's Adventure in Wonderland*. London: MacMillan Company.

quantity rather than the theoretical mathematical negative quantity and will order 1 cubic ft of concrete rather than –1 cubic ft. Absolute value is the positive value of any number (whether it is negative or positive). It is indicated by a vertical mark on both sides of the value (Exhibit 6-6).

Absolute value is indicated by vertical marks:

$|-7| = 7$

$|+7| = 7$

$|+7 \text{ mg}| = 7 \text{ mg}$

$|-7 \text{ mg}| = 7 \text{ mg}$

Exhibit 6-6 Absolute Value

THE 24-HOUR CLOCK

Many institutions record times based on a 24-hour clock. The 24-hour clock records the hours of the day from 1 to 24 rather than the 1 to 12 AM/PM method most clinicians recognize. The advantage of the 24-hour clock is there is greater clarity in distinguishing between an AM (morning) time and a PM (evening) time. Timing on the 24-hour clock requires the addition of 12 to any PM time. So 3:00 PM, for example, becomes 1500 hours. This is pronounced "fifteen hundred hours." Midnight becomes either 2400 (twenty-four hundred hours) or 0000 (zero hours).

Morning times are minimally affected by the 24-hour clock. For example, 8:00 AM is still 0800. This is pronounced "eight hundred hours."

THE SYRINGE

The syringe (Figure 6-1) is used to administer injected medications. Syringes have graduated marks etched on the cylinder, a **plunger** to push the medication out, and a detachable needle to penetrate the patient's skin.

Most syringes are graduated in milliliters or tenths of milliliters. A special 1 ml syringe, used for administering insulin, may be graduated in units.

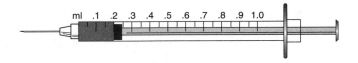

Figure 6-1 1 ml Insulin Syringe

A clinician who has calculated the correct amount of medication to administer may become confused by the graduations on the syringe. For example, a clinician who must give 6.5 ml of medication may draw up exactly that amount. The 6.5 ml will fill the syringe to the 6.5 ml mark. The clinician simply gives the entire amount.

Some medications are supplied in prefilled syringes. For example, if the clinician has calculated that 6.5 ml must be given and the medication is supplied in a prefilled 10 ml syringe, to what graduation mark must the plunger be pushed to administer the correct amount? In this case the syringe is graduated from the needle side at zero to the plunger side at 10 ml. Therefore, to calculate the mark at which the plunger must be stopped, the clinician must subtract the calculated dose from the total in the syringe, as shown in Exhibit 6-8.

To calculate the mark at which the plunger must be stopped, subtract the dose volume from the total volume of the syringe.

Exhibit 6-7 Syringe Rule

Physician order: give 6.5 ml from a 10.0 ml syringe

Unknown: at what mark the plunger should stop

x = (total med in syringe) − (dose)

x = 10.0 ml − 6.5 ml

x = 3.5 ml mark on the syringe

Exhibit 6-8 Example of the Syringe Rule

The same rule can be applied to subsequent administrations of medication from the same syringe. For example, a patient who receives 5 ml of morphine from a 10 ml syringe and 10 minutes later receives an additional 5 ml can have the syringe rule applied to each dose. In the first dose, the total medication is 10 ml. In the second dose, it is only 5 ml.

TOTAL DAILY DOSE

It may be necessary for a clinician to figure the individual dose based on a total daily dose and the number of doses given in a day. An order may be stated like "give 1 g a day in 4 doses," as the example in Exhibit 6-9 does. The medication may be a tablet, intravenous infusion, or injectable medicine.

Give 1 g in 4 doses over 24 hours. Each pill is 125 mg. What is the individual dose, and how many pills are taken?

$$\frac{x}{1 \text{ dose}} = \frac{1 \text{ g}}{4 \text{ doses}}$$

Step 1: We set up an equation to solve for the metric dose.

$x = 250$ mg

$$\frac{x}{250 \text{ mg}} = \frac{1 \text{ pill}}{125 \text{ mg}}$$

Step 2: We set up an equation to solve for the number of pills in the metric dose.

$x = 2$ pills

Exhibit 6-9 Example Total Daily Dose

The total daily dose may also be calculated from the number of individual doses and the frequency of doses. This calculation is often made to prevent an inadvertent overdose.

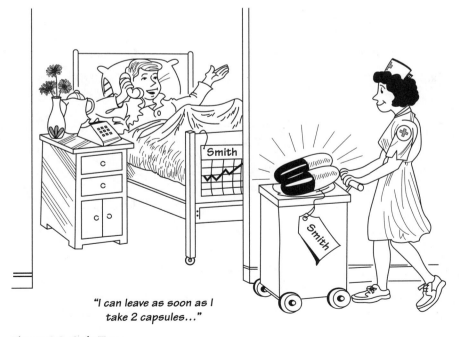

"I can leave as soon as I take 2 capsules..."

Figure 6-2 Only Two

REVIEW PROBLEMS

1. A prefilled syringe contains 100 mg of a medication in 10 ml. The physician orders 60 mg to be administered. The clinician will stop the syringe's plunger at the _____ mark.

Use the following information to solve problems 2–3. A patient requires only 50% of the normal dose of lidocaine. The normal dose is 85 mg. The medication is supplied in 5 ml/100 mg concentration.

2. How many milligrams does the patient receive? _____
3. How many milliliters will be injected? _____
4. An order is given to administer metronidazole in an 8 mg/ml concentration. The medication is supplied in a vial as a powder of 500 mg concentration. What should the total milliliters be to give the desired concentration? _____
5. In Problem 4, 4.4 ml of sterile water was required to reconstitute the metronidazole, giving a concentration of 500 mg/5 ml. How much of that medicine should be added to a 250 ml container to achieve the concentration of 8 mg/ml? _____
6. How much medication is added to a 500 ml IV solution to achieve the concentration of 8 mg/ml? _____

Complete the following table.

	Number	Percent	Decimal
Ex.	$3/5$	60%	0.6
	$2/8$	7. _____	8. _____
	$3^1/_3$	9. _____	10. _____
	11. _____	50%	12. _____
	13. _____	14. _____	0.67
	$13/15$	15. _____	16. _____
	$5/3$	17. _____	18. _____

Number	**Percent**	**Decimal**
$^3/_5$	19. _____	20. _____
$^{15}/_{90}$	21. _____	22. _____
23. _____	90%	24. _____
25. _____	175%	26. _____
27. _____	250%	28. _____

Determine the absolute values.

29. $|6|$ = _____   30. $|-6|$ = _____

31. $|0.75|$ = _____   32. $|-0.75|$ = _____

33. $|8|$ = _____   34. $|-8|$ = _____

35. $|0|$ = _____   36. $|-0|$ = _____

Use the following information to solve problems 37–40. A syringe came pre-filled with 10 ml of a 1% solution of lidocaine. It was used on a patient. The plunger now rests at the 3.5 ml mark.

37. How many milliliters were given? _____

38. How many milligrams were given? _____

39. The physician orders an additional dose of half the original dose. Does this syringe contain sufficient medication to administer the second dose? _____

40. How many milliliters does the second dose require? _____

Convert the following times to times on the 24-hour clock.

41. 7:00 AM _____   42. 7:00 PM _____

43. 10:00 AM _____   44. 10:00 PM _____

45. 12:00 AM _____   46. 12:00 PM _____

47. A vial of medication contains 1 g of medicine in 15 ml. How many milliliters contains 50 mg? _____

48. Define reconstitution.

   _____

   _____

   _____

49. Where may the clinician always find the concentration of a medication?

   _____

   _____

   _____

50. Define absolute value.

   _____

   _____

   _____

Chapter 7

Titration Calculations

I like to take in hand none but clean, virgin fair-and-square mathematical jobs, something that regularly begins at the beginning, and is at the middle when midway, and comes to an end at the conclusion.

—Herman Melville, *Moby Dick.*

Exhibit 7-1

OBJECTIVES

Upon completion of this chapter the clinician should be able to:

1. Given a starting mass of medication, calculate the amount of water to be added to the medicine to create the concentration ordered
2. Given either the percent by mass or percent by volume of medicine, calculate the amount of water to add to an existing concentration to create a new concentration
3. After calculating a new concentration, use the ordered mass to calculate the related volume of medication to be given
4. After calculating a new concentration, use the ordered volume to calculate the related mass of medication to be given

KEY TERMS

dilution
mixture
Mixture Rule

titration
variable

TITRATION

A medication **titration** changes the concentration of a medication by adding a known amount of a solvent (usually water) until a change occurs. This creates a new concentration (mass of medication per unit of volume) by changing the volume. The new concentration must be used for calculating the dose of medication to be given. Once the new concentration has been determined, the problem becomes a standard concentration problem, as discussed in Chapter 5.

A concentration is always composed of two components: a medication and a solvent. Changes in concentration represent a change in the volume of the solvent or, less frequently, a change in the mass of medication. A careful approach to setting up these concentration problems makes them easier to understand and manage.

The mass of medication usually remains constant, and the clinician changes the concentration to a weaker solution by adding more solvent. Concentration problems involving a **dilution** to a weaker concentration always require adding more solvent to the **mixture**.

Some medications are injurious to the body when concentrated. These medications are diluted to make them less injurious. For example, it is common to dilute intravenous medications given to infants because their systems are more sensitive to some concentrated medications than adults are.

Concentration problems requiring a dilution to a weaker (smaller percent) concentration are solved by adding more solvent to the mixture.

Exhibit 7-2 Concentration Mixture

The solvent may be sterile water, a dextrose 5% in water (D5W) solution, or even blood. It does not matter what the solvent is for the purpose of dosage calculation, as long as the solvent is not another active medication. For purposes of calculation, this text will consider all solvents to be sterile water.

MIXTURE RULE

The **Mixture Rule** states that the titration is *always* equal to the sum of the medication and the water.

---

medication + water = new titration (concentration)

Exhibit 7-3 Mixture Rule

The Mixture Rule can be used to calculate the volume or percent of any one of its parts if the volume or percent of the other two parts is known. The percent of the new titration is always 100% because it is the new whole (100%) mixture.

The percent of the new titration is *always* 100%.

Exhibit 7-4 New Titration Concentration

In Exhibit 7-5 and Exhibit 7-6, a medication of 1 ml is mixed to a concentration of 10 ml. The medication is 10% of the mixture.

---

medication + water = new titration

10% + w = 100%

10% + w − 10% = 100% − 10%

w = 90%

Exhibit 7-5 Example Calculation of Percent Water

The volume of the new titration is 10 ml; the volume of the water may be calculated using the Mixture Rule.

---

medication + water = new titration

1 ml + w = 10 ml

1 ml + w − 1 ml = 10 ml − 1 ml

w = 9 ml

Exhibit 7-6 Example Calculation of Water Volume

The Mixture Rule may also be used to calculate the medication part. In Exhibit 7-7, a medication is mixed to a concentration of 10 ml. Because the clinician knows that the volume of the water is 9 ml and the volume of the new titration is 10 ml, the volume of the medication may be calculated.

medication + water = new titration

$m + 9$ ml = 10 ml

$m + 9$ ml − 9 ml = 10 ml − 9 ml

$m = 1$ ml

Exhibit 7-7 Example Calculation of Medication Volume

In Exhibit 7-8, morphine sulphate is supplied in a 1 ml ampule containing 15 mg of medication. Titrate (i.e., mix) this to a concentration of 1 mg/ml. This problem is recognized as a concentration problem because it is using a mass/volume expression. The objective is to determine how much water will be added to the medication given. If the total volume is known, the amount of water may be calculated using the Mixture Rule. The new total volume (t) may be calculated using a concentration ratio equation. Step 1 is to determine the total volume of the mixture based on the new stated concentration, as shown in Exhibit 7-8.

$$\frac{t}{15 \text{ mg}} = \frac{1 \text{ ml}}{1 \text{ mg}}$$

$$\frac{(15 \text{ mg})t}{15 \text{ mg}} = \frac{1 \text{ ml}(15 \text{ mg})}{1 \text{ mg}}$$

$$t = 15 \text{ ml}$$

t represents the total volume of the new titration.

Exhibit 7-8 Example Titration Calculation

Step 2 is to calculate the amount of water (w) in the mixture. The Mixture Rule is used in the example in Exhibit 7-9.

medication + water = new titration

med + water (− med) = new titration (−med)

water (med − med) = new titration (−med)

water = new titration − medication

w = 15 ml − 1 ml

w = 14 ml

Exhibit 7-9 Calculating Water to Be Added

PERCENT

Percent concentration problems may be confusing because there are several factors in the problem. A chart displaying the known data is convenient for organizing the data. Such a chart also is helpful for setting up an equation. A chart may be structured with referenced data across the top, and medication, water, and new titration down the left side.

	%	Mass	Volume	Concentration
Medication	known	known	known	known mass initial volume
Water	x	not applicable	w	not applicable
(New) titration	100%	same as medication above	v (w + medication volume)	known mass (new) volume

Exhibit 7-10 Mixture Chart Template

The chart in Exhibit 7-10 sets up a format to organize the given data and place it in a parallel written format. Information that is given in a problem can be put in the appropriate block. The other blocks may be labeled "unknown" and may be calculated, if needed. This chart accomplishes the first two steps of word problems: identifying what is unknown/asked for and identifying what is known. The new titration is always 100%. Water has no mass of medication or final concentration (unless medication is added), so those blocks in the chart are not applicable.

The example in Exhibit 7-11 demonstrates how the clinician can calculate the amount of water to add to 1 g of a medication to form a mixture solution of 1 mg/ml. This is a concentration problem studied in earlier chapters, and it can be solved using the standard concentration set-up. In this example it is approached as part of a series of calculations. The answer is then used to help fill in the chart and to subsequently calculate other parts of the chart. An equation may be set up by taking any unknown and its related, known reference as well as 2 known references in a parallel column. (The other references may be either a vertical or a horizontal parallel column.) This gives 3 known references to use to set up an equation. Exhibit 7-11 demonstrates how to use the chart to set up an equation. The chart can be used to find how much water (w) must be added or what the ending volume (v) will be. Again, any two parallel items on the chart may be used as a ratio. Exhibit 7-11 uses a medication that is supplied in a 1 g vial with a volume of 30 ml to make a new concentration of 1 mg/ml.

The doctor orders a medication to be mixed to a 1 mg/ml concentration. The medication is supplied in a 1 g/30 ml vial.

	%	Mass	Volume	Concentration
Medication	unknown	1 g	30 ml	$\dfrac{1\ g}{30\ ml}$
Water	unknown	not applicable	w	not applicable
(New) titration	100%	1 g	v	$\dfrac{1\ mg}{1\ ml}$

w in this chart represents the amount of water to be added. The given concentration is 1 g/30 ml. The ordered concentration is 1 mg/ml. v equals the total volume of the new concentration.

Using the concentration set-up, one can solve for v (the volume of the concentration):

$$\frac{v}{1\ g} = \frac{1\ ml}{1\ mg}$$

$v = 1{,}000$ ml (or 1 L)

The volume includes both water and medication. The medication has a volume of 30 ml. Remembering that $v = m + w$ (volume = medication + water), the clinician can now set up the equation to solve for the amount of water to be used.

$v = m + w$

$1{,}000$ ml $= 30$ ml $+ w$

$w = 1{,}000$ ml $- 30$ ml

$w = 970$ ml   (For practical purposes, most clinicians won't bother to draw 30 ml out of a liter IV solution because the difference is not significant.)

Exhibit 7-11 Example Concentration Problem Chart

In the example in Exhibit 7-12, the clinician must calculate how much water (w) to add to a mixture to dilute the medication to a 50% concentration. Horizontally parallel items are used to establish a ratio equation in the following manner. The unknown volume of the titration is related to the known percent (100%) of the titration. The water line of the chart has no known values to work with, so we must use two steps to calculate the amount of water to be added. The first step is to determine the concentration of the water. The second step is to use the concentration to set up a ratio equation to solve for the volume of water (w). The parallel ratio is used to relate the known volume of medication to the known percent of the mixture.

The medication is provided in a 50 ml container. The doctor wants it diluted to a 50% concentration before administration. How much water is to be added?

	%	Mass	Volume	Concentration
Medication	50%	known	50 ml	known mass / initial volume
Water	x	not applicable	w	not applicable
(New) titration	100%	same as medication above	unknown	known mass / new volume

How much water is to be added to dilute the medication to 50%? There is no value on the water line to use for calculation, so we must first solve for a value and then, as a second step, use a simple ratio equation to solve for the volume of water (w).

Remembering that the total volume = medication + water, the equation can be set up as:

100% = 50% + x

x = 50%

The clinician has determined that 50% of the mixture should be water. The second step is to solve for the volume of water.

$$\frac{w}{50\%} = \frac{50 \text{ ml (med)}}{50\%}$$

w = 50 ml

Exhibit 7-12 Example Mixture Problem

The example in Exhibit 7-13 demonstrates how the clinician can use the medication concentration to calculate the total volume of the new concentration. Vertically parallel items are used to establish a ratio equation. A clinician would need to know this to set up an IV titration with the proper volume IV solution. The unknown volume of the titration is related to the known volume of medication. The parallel ratio relates the known percent (100%)

of the titration to the known percent of medication. The use of the chart format visually reinforces the equation set-up.

The medication is provided in a 25 ml container. The doctor wants it diluted to a 10% concentration before administration. How much water is to be added? What size IV container is needed?

	%	Mass	Volume	Concentration
Medication	10%	known	25 ml	$\dfrac{\text{unknown mass}}{\text{25 ml}}$
Water	x	not applicable	w	not applicable
(New) titration	100%	same as medication above	unknown	$\dfrac{\text{unknown mass}}{v}$

There is no value on the water line to use for calculation, so we must first solve for a percent value and then, as a second step, use a simple ratio equation to solve for the volume of water (w).

Remembering that the total volume = medication + water, the equation can be set up as:

$100\% = 10\% + x$

$x = 90\%$

The clinician has determined that 90% of the mixture should be water. The second step is to solve for the volume of water.

$$\frac{w}{90\%} = \frac{25\text{ ml (med)}}{10\%}$$

$w = 225$ ml   A 250 ml IV solution would be appropriate. To be precise, a clinician could waste 25 ml of a 250 ml IV solution and add the medication.

Exhibit 7-13 Example Volume Problem

The example in Exhibit 7-14 demonstrates how the clinician may solve for the new total volume and select the correctly sized syringe to administer the medication. There are several unknowns. x represents the percent of water. w represents the volume of water. v represents the total volume. These different symbols are used rather than repeating the standard unknown symbol, x, to clarify what is being calculated and to try to reduce possible confusion between the unknown **variables**; this way the x symbol is used only once. Analysis of the question indicates it asks for w, the volume of water added.

The clinician may use any symbol to represent an unknown. It is wise to avoid using characters that might be confused with abbreviations, such as g for gram or L for liter.

A medication is supplied in a 10 mg/ml vial. The doctor ordered it mixed to a 10% concentration and administered as an IV bolus. How much *water* is added? What is the most convenient size syringe to use?

	%	Mass	Volume	Concentration
Medication	10%	10 mg	1 ml	$\dfrac{10\ mg}{ml}$
Water	x	not applicable	w	not applicable
(New) titration	100%	same as medication above	v	$\dfrac{10\ mg}{v}$

There is no value on the water line to use for calculation, so we must first solve for a percent value and then, as a second step, use a simple ratio equation to solve for the volume of water (w).

Remembering that the total volume = medication + water, the equation can be set up as:

$100\% = 10\% + x$

$x = 90\%$

The clinician has determined that 90% of the mixture should be water. The second step is to solve for the volume of water.

$$\frac{w}{90\%} = \frac{1\ ml\ (med)}{10\%}$$

$w = 9$ ml   A 10 ml syringe would hold both medication and solvent. The volume of the medication is 10% of the solution and is significant to the mixture and should be included in calculations.

Exhibit 7-14 Example Volume Problem

The clinician can use the calculated value for the water added to calculate the total volume and concentration, as demonstrated in Exhibit 7-15. Once the volume of the titration (v) is calculated, the new concentration (c) can be calculated. The new concentration is the mass of the medication divided by the new total volume (v). The mass of the medication is not altered by adding water. Therefore, the concentration is the existing mass divided by the new total concentration.

	%	Mass	Volume	Concentration
Medication	10%	10 mg	1 ml	10 mg/ml
Water	90%	(none)	9 ml	(none)
(New) titration	100%	10 mg	v	c

Once the volume of water added is calculated, the clinician can use the Mixture Rule to calculate the total volume and the concentration.

volume = medication + Water

$v = 9$ ml + 1 ml

$v = 10$ ml

$c = 10$ mg/10 ml or 1 mg/ml

Exhibit 7-15 Example Titration Calculation

The ratio equation can be set up to solve for the amount of water or the total volume as long as the percent is known (Exhibit 7-16).

$$\frac{w}{90\%} = \frac{1\ ml}{10\%} \qquad \text{or} \qquad \frac{t}{100\%} = \frac{1\ ml}{10\%}$$

$$w = 9\ ml \qquad\qquad\qquad t = 10\ ml$$

Exhibit 7-16 Example Mixture Problem

PREPARATION OF NEW SOLUTIONS

The percent of a solution represents the number of milliliters of medication per total volume (in milliliters) of the mixed solution as indicated in Exhibit 7-17. This preparation is rarely required of a health care provider. However, it may be necessary to calculate the volume or number of grams of medication received from a solution. D5W is dextrose 5% in water. This is a concentration of 5 g of dextrose in 100 ml of sterile water. One percent lidocaine represents 1 ml of lidocaine in 100 ml of solution.

$$\text{Percent of solution} = \frac{\text{(ml of medication)}100\%}{\text{ml (total volume of solution)}}$$

$$\text{Example} = \frac{\text{(10 ml medication)}100\%}{\text{50 ml (total volume of solution)}}$$

$$= \frac{1{,}000\%}{50}$$

$$= 20\%$$

Exhibit 7-17 Example Percent Problem

Titration problems may be confusing because there are many data elements to manage. The key to simplifying the problem set-up is to have an organized approach to the problem. Once the titration has been established, the problem becomes a standard concentration problem. The Mixture Rule helps simplify the equation when all that is needed is the percent or volume of water to add.

REVIEW PROBLEMS

1. Sodium bicarbonate is commonly supplied in a 50 ml prefilled syringe containing 50 mEq. Dilute this to a 50% concentration, and administer 35 mEq. How much of the titration does the clinician administer? _____

Complete the concentration chart in Exhibit 7-18 based on problem 1.

	%	Mass	Volume	Concentration
Medication	2. _____	3. _____	4. _____	5. _____
Water	6. _____	7. _____	8. _____	(none)
(New)	100%	9. _____	10. _____	11. _____

Exhibit 7-18 Review Problems 2–11

12. Epinephrine may be supplied in a concentration of 1/1,000 containing 1 mg in 1 ml. Mix this to a 10% solution, and administer 0.5 mg. How much of the titration does the clinician administer? _____

Complete the concentration chart in Exhibit 7-19 based on problem 12.

	%	Mass	Volume	Concentration
Medication	13. _____	14. _____	15. _____	16. _____
Water	17. _____	18. _____	19. _____	(none)
(New) titration	100%	20. _____	21. _____	22. _____

Exhibit 7-19 Review Problems 13–22

23. Lidocaine may be supplied in a 1% solution containing 0.1 g in 10 ml. If a clinician received a 2% solution instead of a 1% solution, it would contain _____ in 10 ml.
24. If the clinician were ordered to administer 85 mg of the 2% lidocaine supplied in Problem 4, how many milliliters would be given? _____
25. Calcium chloride may be supplied in a solution containing 1 g in 10 ml. If the clinician dilutes this to one-half strength, how much water will be added? _____

Complete the concentration chart in Exhibit 7-20 based on problem 25.

	%	Mass	Volume	Concentration
Medication	26. _____	27. _____	28. _____	29. _____
Water	30. _____	31. _____	32. _____	(none)
(New) titration	100%	33. _____	34. _____	35. _____

Exhibit 7-20 Review Problems 26–35

36. Dextrose 50% in water (D50W) is commonly supplied in a 50 ml syringe. If the clinician is ordered to dilute this concentration to D25W, how much water will be added? _____
37. Lidocaine may be supplied as 1 g in 30 ml. If the clinician wished to administer a bolus of 50 mg in a concentration of 10 mg/ml, how many milliliters of lidocaine will he use if he draws up only the required dose of 50 mg? _____

Complete the concentration chart in Exhibit 7-21 using the following information. Dr. Einstein ordered 5 mg of morphine sulphate, titrated to a 1 mg/ml solution, to be administered to a patient. The morphine is supplied in a 1 ml vial containing 15 mg of medication.

	%	Mass	Volume	Concentration
Medication	38. _____	39. _____	40. _____	41. _____
Water	42. _____	43. _____	44. _____	(none)
(New) titration	100%	45. _____	46. _____	47. _____

Exhibit 7-21 Review Problems 38–47

48. A clinician mixes 9 ml of water with 1 ml of morphine (15 mg/ml) and administers 5 ml of the new mixture, how much morphine is being given? _____
49. If the clinician in Problem 48 wanted to dilute the titration to a 10% solution, how much more water should be added? _____
50. Define titration.

_____

_____

_____

Chapter 8

Infusions, Concentrations, and Drip Rate Calculations

> Words are acoustical signs for concepts; concepts, however, are more or less definite image signs for often recurring and associated sensations, for groups of sensations. To understand one another, it is not enough that one use the same words; one also has to use the same words for the same species of inner experiences.
>
> —Friedrich Nietzsche.

Exhibit 8-1

OBJECTIVES

Upon completion of this chapter the clinician should be able to:

1. Calculate the amount of medication required for a volume of fluid to get to a desired concentration
2. Calculate units of volume from given units of mass of medication
3. Convert between units of hours, days, and minutes
4. Convert between units of liters, milliliters, and drops
5. Calculate drip rates of IV infusion and express them in drops per minute
6. Given an IV flow rate, calculate how long a volume of solution will last

KEY TERMS

colloid	isotonic
crystalloid	KVO
flow rate	solute
hypertonic	solvent
hypotonic	

INTRAVENOUS MEDICATION

Many medications are given intravenously. The intravenous route has many advantages, as discussed in Chapter 1. Intravenous medications must be closely controlled. Medications that are given in a time frame of hours rather than minutes are measured in milliliters per hour and drops (gtt) per minute. The drip rates are administered in the related drops per minute.

SOLUTIONS

A solution is a mixture of a solvent and a solute. The **solvent** is the fluid medium into which the solute is dissolved. The **solute** is the ingredient that is added to the solvent.

Solutions are classified by their relative concentrations. A concentration that is more concentrated than human blood serum is **hypertonic**. A hypertonic solution has a greater osmotic pressure than human cells. This pressure will allow water to osmose from human cells into an area of hypertonicity. This will dehydrate the body and may cause volume overload in the vascular system.

A solution less concentrated than human blood serum is **hypotonic**. A hypotonic solution has an osmotic pressure less than that of human cells or fluids. This pressure will allow water to osmose from a hypotonic solution into human fluids and then into human cells. This will cause the body to develop fluid overload with possible pulmonary edema.

A solution that has the same concentration of solutes as human blood is **isotonic**. An isotonic solution has 0.9% solutes dissolved. An isotonic solution has the same osmotic pressure as human cells and fluids and will cause no fluid shift in an otherwise healthy patient.

A **crystalloid** solution has solutes that have completely dissolved in it. It will diffuse through animal membranes, such as a cell wall. Most solutes capable of dissolving in solution are crystalline.

A **colloid** solution holds large molecules, such as human proteins. These large molecules will not completely dissolve. This solution will not diffuse through a cell wall because of the size of the suspended particles. A colloid is not scientifically a true solution because the solutes do not completely dissolve. Human blood is a tissue and an example of a colloidal solution.

Popular solutions for medical purposes include lactated Ringers, normal (0.9% sodium chloride) saline, and D5W (dextrose 5% in water). Normal saline is called "normal" because it is isotonic and has the same concentration of solutes as human blood.

INFUSION CALCULATIONS

IV infusions present two types of calculation problems, which are related. Concentration of medication in the IV solution is one type of problem. The other is determining flow rate. These are easily distinguished because a concentration involves mass per unit of volume and rate involves volume per unit of time.

CONCENTRATION PROBLEMS

Concentration problems are very similar to those studied in previous chapters. In Exhibit 8-2, an order is given to mix a lidocaine infusion solution with a concentration of 2 mg/ml. This exhibit shows how the clinician may calculate the volume of 2 mg/ml for this concentration.

Problem: Give 4 mg/min.

Unknown: How many milliliters is 4 mg.

Known: The medication concentration is 1 mg/ml, or 4 g/L.

$$\frac{x}{-} = \frac{}{\rule{2cm}{0.4pt}}$$

$$\frac{x}{4 \text{ mg}} = \frac{1 \text{ ml}}{1 \text{ mg}}$$

$$x = \frac{1 \text{ ml}}{1 \text{ mg}} (4 \text{ mg})$$

$$x = 4 \text{ ml}$$

Exhibit 8-2 Sample Concentration Problem

The addition of 4 g to a 1-liter solution will increase the volume of the solution from 1 liter to 1 liter 10 ml. The additional volume of medication is considered insignificant for most administrations of 250 ml or more. It usually does not require a recalculation to account for a total volume of 1,010 ml. Smaller containers or syringes may require the recalculation of the concentration.

Many infusion orders are expressed as mass per unit of time, which must be converted to units of volume per unit of time to calculate the IV drip rate. This is the type of concentration problem addressed in Chapter 5 of this text. The clinician is ordered to give 2 ml/min and must calculate how many drops should be flowed over a minute (Exhibit 8-3).

Problem:	Convert milliliters to drops for IV rate of 2 ml/min.
Unknown:	How many drops are in 2 ml.
Known:	The package label states that there are 60 gtt/ml (60 drops per milliliter)

$$\frac{x}{2} = \frac{}{}$$

$$\frac{x}{2 \text{ ml}} = \frac{60 \text{ gtt}}{1 \text{ ml}}$$

$$x = \frac{60 \text{ gtt} \ (2 \text{ ml})}{1 \text{ ml}}$$

$$x = 120 \text{ gtt}$$

Exhibit 8-3 Example IV Infusion Calculation

IV SET-UPS

IV infusions are regulated by visual adjustment of an inline flow meter in the IV tubing (Figure 8-1) or by using an IV pump. The IV set-up, like the syringe, measures volume rather than mass of medication. It measures volume in a see-through drip chamber in which the drops may be counted. The flow meter permits the clinician to adjust the flow to regulate the drops. The clinician may need to calculate drops per minute from an order stated in milliliters per hour to correctly adjust the flow rate.

The IV administration set-up will have printed on its package label the unit conversion factor for converting milliliters to drops. There is a variety of drop sizes. Most standard is a unit that has 60 drops per milliliter. Others have 10, 20, or 30 drops per milliliter. Milliliters are converted to drops with the unit conversion factor method. Refer to Exhibit 8-3 as an example.

FLOW RATES

The **flow rate** is a calculation of units of volume per unit of time. The flow rate is sometimes given in an order as milliliters per hour. It is not practical to measure milliliters per hour. If the flow rate were incorrect, the patient could be improperly dosed before the flow rate could be adjusted. The flow rate is converted to a measurable unit of drops per minute. This conversion is accomplished with the unit conversion factor of drops per milliliter, given by the manufacturer of the IV delivery line.

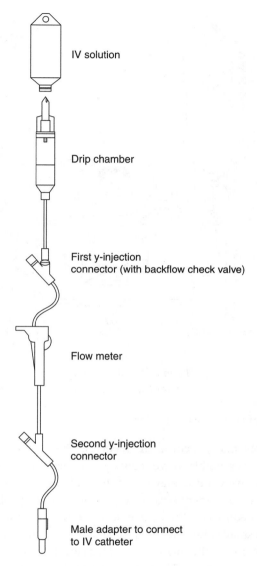

IV solution

Drip chamber

First y-injection
connector (with backflow check valve)

Flow meter

Second y-injection
connector

Male adapter to connect
to IV catheter

Figure 8-1 Sample IV Set-Up

The y-intersection sites allow injection of medication or connection (with a needle) of a second
IV solution. The flow meter adjust drip rate by restricting flow.

KVO/TKO FLOW RATE

IV lines are established for two general purposes. One purpose is to provide an
access route to central circulation to administer medications. This access route
is frequently established as a precaution in patients who have undiagnosed

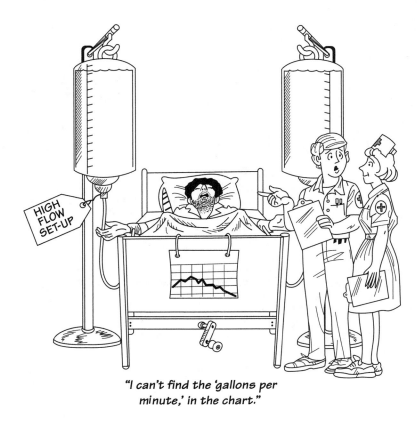

"I can't find the 'gallons per minute,' in the chart."

Figure 8-2 Infusion Rate Calculation

medical problems or medical emergencies. The rate of flow is sometimes set to be as slow as possible to avoid giving unnecessary volume. The administration of excessive volume may result in fluid overload or pulmonary edema and can cause the patient serious respiratory or renal problems. Patients with preexisting medical conditions may suffer these consequences with surprising rapidity and small volumes of fluid. The set-up requires a steady drip to prevent clotting of blood at the incision site. This flow rate is called "keep vein open" (**KVO**) or "to keep open" (TKO). The actual volume infused is about 30 ml/hr.

The other purpose for establishing IV access is to provide fluid for resuscitation. Persons needing fluid, such as shock victims, benefit most from whole blood. These persons should receive an IV with a special set-up device that allows for large drops. This device is frequently called a "blood set." The diameter of the intravenous catheter can reduce the maximum flow rate if a small or long catheter is used. Patients needing volume resuscitation should have a catheter no smaller than an 18 gauge to allow large volumes of fluid to be given as needed.

FLOW RATE RULE

The Flow Rate Rule (Exhibit 8-4) is a method of calculating drops per minute using the unit conversion factor in a substitution method. It multiplies the milliliters per minute by the drops per milliliter to get drops per minute. If the time factor is expressed in a unit other than minutes, it may be converted to minutes using common time unit conversion factors.

$$\frac{\text{milliliters}}{\text{minute}} * \frac{\text{drops}}{\text{milliliter}} = \frac{\text{drops}}{\text{minute}}$$

Exhibit 8-4 Flow Rate Rule

Occasionally, flow rate is expressed as a mass per unit of time, such as 4 mg/min. This flow rate will vary depending on the concentration of the solution. The clinician may choose to make a more concentrated solution for a patient who may be injured by excessive volumes. To calculate a measurable flow rate, this mass must first be converted to a volume using the solution's concentration. Then the drop rate is determined using the Flow Rate Rule, as shown in the example in Exhibit 8-5.

A physician orders a lidocaine infusion of 2 mg/min to be delivered KVO.

The lidocaine is supplied in 2 g/5 ml vials.

The IV set-up delivers 60 gtt/ml.

The IV solution is a 250 ml container.

The first step in this problem is to calculate the concentration. KVO is 30 ml/hr, or 0.5 ml/min. The order is for 2 mg/min. The order is then known to be 2 mg/0.5 ml.

$$\frac{x}{250 \text{ ml}} = \frac{2 \text{ mg}}{0.5 \text{ ml}}$$

$$x = 1{,}000 \text{ mg} = 1 \text{ g}$$

This mass is used to calculate how much lidocaine must be added to the IV solution to yield the correct concentration for the physician's order.

The KVO rate is 30 ml/hr, or 0.5 ml/min. This must be converted to drops per minute. The Flow Rate Rule is convenient for this. A ratio equation may also be used.

$$\text{FR (flow rate)} = \frac{0.5 \text{ ml}}{1 \text{ min}} * \frac{60 \text{ gtt}}{1 \text{ ml}}$$

$$\text{FR} = 30 \text{ gtt/min}$$

Exhibit 8-5 Example Drop Rate Calculation

IV DURATION

A variation of the Flow Rate Rule is used to calculate how long an IV solution will last before requiring replacement. This is a ratio proportion problem that relates volume per unit of time. See Exhibit 8-6 for an example.

A patient has an IV flowing at 30 ml/hr. The solution is a 0.5 L container.

How long will the solution last?

Known: There is 500 ml of solution; Flow rate is 30 ml/hr.

Unknown: How many hours will the solution last?

$$\frac{x}{500 \text{ ml}} = \frac{1 \text{ hr}}{30 \text{ ml}}$$

$$x = \frac{1 \text{ hr} \ (500 \text{ ml})}{30 \text{ ml}}$$

$$x = 16.7 \text{ hr}$$

Exhibit 8-6 Example Flow Rate Calculation

REVIEW PROBLEMS

For problems 1–43, use 60 gtt/ml as the unit conversion factor for the following orders, unless another unit conversion factor is specified.

Mix a concentration of 4 mg/ml in 250 ml and give 2 mg/min. What is the concentration of the infusion?

1. _____ mg/ml   2. _____ g/250 ml

What is the flow rate?

3. _____ ml/min   4. _____ gtt/min

Mix 1 mg in 500 ml and give 2.0 mcg/kg/hr to a 132 lb patient. What is the concentration of the infusion?

5. _____ mcg/ml   6. _____ mg/500 ml

What is the flow rate?

7. _____ ml/min   8. _____ gtt/min

Give a KVO rate (30 ml/hr). Mix a concentration that will deliver 240 mg in the hour. What is the concentration of the infusion?

9. _____ mg/ml   10. _____ g/500 ml

What is the flow rate?

11. _____ ml/min   12. _____ gtt/min

Mix a concentration of 4 mcg/ml in 250 ml and give 6 mcg/min. What is the concentration of the infusion?

13. _____ mcg/ml   14. _____ mg/250 ml

What is the flow rate?

15. _____ ml/min   16. _____ gtt/min

Mix 4 g in 500 ml and give 2 mg/kg/hr to a 264 lb patient. What is the concentration of the infusion?

17. _____ mg/ml   18. _____ m/500 ml

What is the flow rate?

19. _____ ml/min   20. _____ gtt/min

Give a KVO rate (30 ml/hr). Mix a concentration that will deliver 60 mg in the hour. What is the concentration of the infusion?

21. _____ mg/ml   22. _____ mg/100 ml

What is the flow rate?

23. _____ ml/min   24. _____ gtt/min

Mix a medication to a 10 mg/ml concentration in 500 ml and give 5 mg/min. What is the concentration of the infusion? (Disregard the volume change created by adding the medication.)

25. _____ mg/ml   26. _____ g/500 ml

What is the flow rate?

27. _____ ml/min   28. _____ gtt/min

What is the flow rate for an order to give 6 L in 24 hours?

29. _____ ml/hr   30. _____ ml/min

31. _____ gtt/min

32. Flow 120 gtt/min until 1 L is infused. How long will the infusion require? _____

33. In 8 hours at a rate of 120 gtt/min, how many milliliters (60 gtt/ml) will be infused? _____

34. Flow 60 gtt/min until a 250 ml bag of D5W is empty. How long will the infusion last? _____

35. At a KVO rate, how long will it take to infuse 1 L? _____

Mix a concentration of 4 mcg/ml in 250 ml. What is the concentration of the infusion?

36. _____ mg/250 ml   37. _____ mcg/ml

38. How much medication (4 mcg/ml) will be infused after 20 minutes at a KVO rate? _____

39. Give a 2 mg/kg/hr dosage to a 220 lb patient. Mix 40 g in 500 ml. What is the concentration of the infusion? _____ mg/ml

40. How much medication will be infused in 30 minutes? _____

41. If 1 ml of an IV solution contains 20 mcg and the clinician wishes to infuse 40 mcg/min, how many milliliters per hour would the clinician infuse? _____

The doctor ordered a 2 mg/ml IV infusion. To achieve that concentration, the clinician will mix:

42. _____ g/500 ml   43. _____ mg/250 ml

Given the following flow rate order and the following drop to milliliter unit conversion factors, calculate the flow rate in drops per minute.

Flow Rate Order	30 gtt/ml	10 gtt/ml
100 ml/hr	44. _____	45. _____
120 ml/hr	46. _____	47. _____
1 L/8 hr	48. _____	49. _____
60 ml/hr	50. _____	

Chapter 9

Formula Calculations

> And it's never clear who's to navigate and who's to steer. So you flounder, drifting ever near the rocks.
>
> —Dan Fogelberg.

Exhibit 9-1

OBJECTIVES

Upon completion of this chapter the clinician should be able to:

1. Identify the percent of body surface affected by a burn using the Rule of Nines and/or the Lund and Browder chart

2. Calculate flow rates for burn patients using the Parkland (Baxter-Moyer) formula

3. Convert temperature readings between Celsius and Fahrenheit units of measure

4. Calculate pediatric dosages using the Broselow Tape, Clark's Rule, Fried's Rule, or Young's Rule

5. Calculate the expected pH using the Henderson–Hasselbalch equation when given the HCO_3^- and the $PaCO_2$ measurements

KEY TERMS

body temperature
boiling point
Fahrenheit
formula
freezing point

patient weight
Rule of Nines
scale
total body surface area

BURN CALCULATIONS

Burn victims are managed with consideration of the severity of their burns. Severity is determined not only by the depth of the burn but also by the size of the burn. The size of a burn is related to the **total body surface area** (TBSA) as a percent value. There are several ways to determine this.

The **Rule of Nines** is a method of rough estimation. It varies according to the size of the patient (i.e., adult, child, or infant). The Rule of Nines (Figure 9-1) assigns 9% to each major section of the body. This method of estimation of body surface is easy to remember and does not require referring to a chart.

A patient can have more than one type of burn and may present with percents of different degrees. For example, the same patient may present with 2% third-degree burns and 18% second-degree burns for a total burn of 20%. Determining whether a burn is major and what treatment protocol to use may depend on a correct estimate of the burn.

A rough guide to estimating body surface is to estimate an area the size of a hand as being approximately 1% of a person's total body surface area.

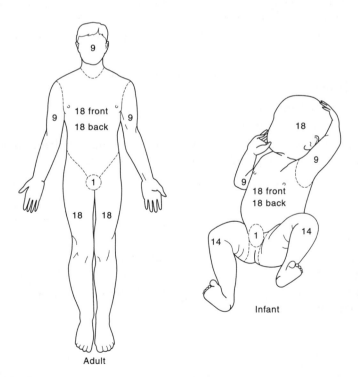

Figure 9-1 Calculating Percent of Burns Based on Rule of Nines: The Most Common Method of Determining Burn Area

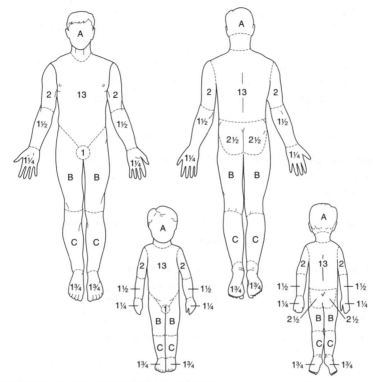

Age (years)	0	1	5	10	15	Adult
A: $\frac{1}{2}$ of head	$9\frac{1}{2}$	$8\frac{1}{2}$	$6\frac{1}{2}$	$5\frac{1}{2}$	$4\frac{1}{2}$	$3\frac{1}{2}$
B: $\frac{1}{2}$ of one thigh	$2\frac{3}{4}$	$3\frac{1}{4}$	4	$4\frac{1}{4}$	$4\frac{1}{2}$	$4\frac{3}{4}$
C: $\frac{1}{2}$ of one leg	$2\frac{1}{2}$	$2\frac{1}{2}$	$2\frac{3}{4}$	3	$3\frac{1}{4}$	3

Figure 9-2 Lund and Browder Chart

LUND AND BROWDER CHART

There are also several professionally developed charts, including the Lund and Browder chart (Figure 9-2), for determining the total body surface area. The percents assigned by the Lund and Browder chart are slightly different from the Rule of Nines.

PARKLAND (BAXTER-MOYER) BURN FORMULA

The Parkland **formula**, originally devised by Dr. Baxter and Dr. Moyer, may be used to calculate flow rates for burns involving 20% to 50% of TBSA but is not reliable for larger burns. Other factors influence flow rates, but this formula can be used as a starting point for intravenous therapy. The Parkland formula (Exhibit 9-2) calculates the total amount of fluid for resuscitation over the first 24 hours. Half of that volume is administered in the first 8 hours, and the other half is given during the last 16 hours. Ongoing burn resuscitation should be guided by other lab values—such as urine flow, hematocrit, and other labs, which are beyond the scope of this text.

For the first 24 hours, the total resuscitation volume is calculated:

$$(4\ ml) * (\text{patient weight in kilograms}) * (\text{TBSA burned}) = \frac{\text{total resuscitation volume}}{24\ hr}$$

Half of the total is given in the first 8 hours:

$$\frac{1}{2} * \frac{\text{total resuscitation volume}}{8\ hr} = \frac{\text{volume}}{hr}$$

The second half is given in the following 16 hours (see Exhibit 9-3 for additional examples):

$$\frac{1}{2} = \frac{\text{total resuscitation volume}}{16\ hr} = \frac{\text{volume}}{hr}$$

Volume per hour must then be converted to drops per minute.

Burn resuscitation is a sophisticated process with many formulas, none of which has demonstrated a clear superiority over the others. Resuscitation should be guided by a set of criteria including urine flow and other values.

Source: Baxter CR. (1974). Fluid Volume and Electrolyte Changes in the Early Post-Burn Period. *Clinics in Plastic Surgery,* 1:643–709.

Exhibit 9-2 Parkland (Baxter-Moyer) Formula

For example, in a burn patient weighing 180 lb with 35% TBSA affected, the formula would be applied as it is in Exhibit 9-3.

In this example of the Parkland Formula:

x is the total volume to be given in the first 24 hours;

y represents the flow rate for the first 8 hours of the first 24 hours; and

z represents the flow rate for the subsequent 16 hours of the first 24 hours.

$$x = 4\ ml * 82\ kg * 35$$
$$x = 11\ \text{liters}\ 480\ ml$$
$$y = \frac{1}{2} * \frac{x}{8\ hr} = \frac{11{,}480\ ml}{16\ hr} = 717.5\ ml/hr$$
$$z = \frac{1}{2} * \frac{x}{16\ hr} = \frac{11{,}480\ ml}{32\ hr} = 359\ ml/hr$$

Exhibit 9-3 Example of the Parkland Formula

TEMPERATURE

The metric system uses temperature readings in degrees Celsius. Clinicians may have patients who report their temperature in **Fahrenheit** (F) or Celsius (C). Medical personnel may need to use scientific instruments calibrated in degrees Celsius. Memorization of a few basic conversion points between Fahrenheit and Celsius, as shown in Exhibit 9-4, will meet most needs.

	Fahrenheit	**Celsius**
Boiling point of water	212°	100°
Normal body temperature	98.6°	37°
Freezing point of water	32°	0°

Exhibit 9-4 Comparison of Fahrenheit to Celsius

Average **body temperature** is 37°C. A patient with a temperature greater than 37°C may have a fever or other temperature disturbance (such as heatstroke). A temperature lower than 37°C is below normal and possibly hypothermia. Human temperature, like many other measurements, may vary slightly without being considered abnormal. The **freezing point** of water is 0°C, and the **boiling point** is 100°C.

Conversion between the two **scales** must first take the starting point of the Celsius scale into account. Otherwise, every degree on the Fahrenheit scale is 5/9 of a Celsius degree. Confusion about which degree is the larger may be reduced by recalling that the freezing and boiling points of water on the Celsius scale are a range of 100° (0–100°C). The same range for the Fahrenheit scale is 180° (32–212°F). The ratio between 100°C and 180°F is shown in Exhibit 9-5.

Celsius : Fahrenheit   100°C:180°F

OR, reduced to the lowest common denominator:

$$\frac{100°C}{20} : \frac{180°F}{20}$$

Celsius : Fahrenheit   5°C:9°F

Exhibit 9-5 Celsius to Fahrenheit Unit Conversion Factor

Conversion from either Celsius or Fahrenheit can use the factor in Exhibit 9-5 (5°C : 9°F) as a unit conversion factor. Before making a unit conversion, the clinician must account for the different starting points of the scales. The starting point for the Celsius scale is 0°C, which is also the freezing point of water. The parallel point, or the freezing point of water, on the Fahrenheit scale is 32°F. The Fahrenheit scale starts 32° higher than the Celsius scale. Conversion to Celsius must begin by subtracting 32° from the beginning Fahrenheit temperature. Conversion to Fahrenheit includes first making the unit conversion and then adding the 32° to the Fahrenheit temperature. Many clinicians have difficulty remembering which conversion requires subtraction and whether that subtraction is performed before or after the unit conversion. It may help to remember that the metric scale is the standard in most of the world. It is the Fahrenheit scale that is scientifically different (i.e., not standard); therefore, the additions or subtractions must all be made on the Fahrenheit scale.

The range from freezing to boiling is 100° on the Celsius scale but 180° on the Fahrenheit scale, so each Celsius unit is a bit larger than each Fahrenheit unit. The clinician would expect, as a general guideline, a lower number on the Celsius scale for a given temperature on the Fahrenheit scale. Conversion from Celsius to Fahrenheit (Exhibit 9-6) is a conversion from a smaller unit to a larger unit. Therefore, the unit conversion factor is 9°F/5°C.

Formula: $\qquad\qquad °C * \dfrac{9°F}{5°C} + 32°F$

Example: Convert 37°C to degrees Fahrenheit

$$37°C * \frac{9°F}{5°C} + 32°F$$

$$66.6°F + 32°F = 98.6°F$$

Exhibit 9-6 Conversion to Fahrenheit

Conversion from Fahrenheit to Celsius (Exhibit 9-7) is a conversion from a larger unit to a smaller unit. The end number of units will be smaller because each individual unit is smaller. Therefore, the unit conversion factor will be 5°C/9°F. If your Celsius temperature is higher than the equivalent Fahrenheit temperature (i.e., for temperatures above 0°C), you made a mistake in your calculation. Remember: the addition or subtraction is always performed on the Fahrenheit scale.

Formula: $(°F - 32) * \dfrac{5°C}{9°F}$

Example: Convert 98.6°F to degrees Celsius

$(98.6°F - 32°F) * \dfrac{5°C}{9°F}$

$66.6°F * \dfrac{5°C}{9°F} = 37°C$

Exhibit 9-7 Conversion to Celsius

PEDIATRIC DOSES AND FORMULAS

Children present special problems for dosage calculations. They often do not tolerate adult doses of medication. The therapeutic envelope for children is narrower than it is for adults because their body masses are smaller and because their systems may be more sensitive to some medications, especially hypertonic medications. Pediatric doses permit very small margins for error, require greater precision than adult doses, and must be most carefully calculated. The use of a unit conversion factor for pounds to kilograms of 2.2 (rounded off from 2.204) may not be precise enough in the preadolescent patient. Calculations are complicated by the inconsistencies in growth rates, weights, and development among children, even those of the same age. The clinician should adhere to pediatric doses published in the *United States Pharmacopeia*. Some doses may be calculated based on body weight. Others may use the West Nomogram (discussed later in this chapter) or factors like patient age. The child who is undergoing chemotherapy may require very special doses.

If a medication does not have a published pediatric dose, the dose must be determined or calculated. There are several methods of dosage determination for children. The methods are named after the persons who developed them. These are the Broselow Tape, Clark's Rule, Fried's Rule, and Young's Rule. The Broselow Tape (Figure 9-3 and Figure 9-4) estimates weight

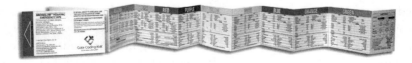

Figure 9-3 The Broselow Tape

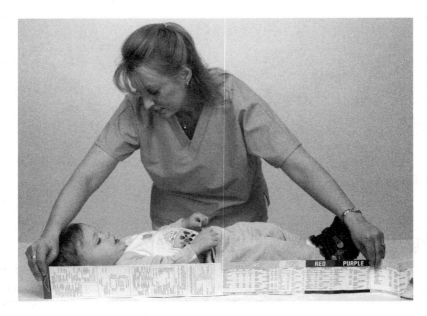

Figure 9-4 The Broselow Pediatric Tape

and dose based on body height. The other rules estimate weight and dose based on patient age. Remember: children who have underlying medical problems or who are undergoing chemotherapy may require very special doses.

Pediatric IV fluid doses are frequently administered through a 100 ml container to avoid accidental fluid overload. The volume of the medication added to a 100 ml container is usually significant and should be considered in calculating the dose or flow rate.

BROSELOW TAPE

A method of determining dose and **patient weight** very quickly and simply is the Broselow Tape. The Broselow Tape is a measuring tape with increments marked in kilograms of weight on one side and color-coded equipment sizes on the other. The tape is used to measure a child from head to foot. The child's weight is determined by length. The correct doses of medications used in emergency resuscitation are indicated on the tape at each size increment. The tape is very reliable. It does tend to underestimate the weight slightly (by about 0.5 kg), but not by a clinically significant amount. It's least accurate in judging the body weight of obese patients (i.e., those 25 kg above their ideal body weight). "The tape also was shown to be significantly more accurate than those weight estimates made from age and observation by residents and pediatric nurses."[1]

Perhaps the principal advantage of the tape is that it eliminates weight calculations completely for children. It also eliminates the need to calculate doses for resuscitation drugs in acute emergencies. And it further eliminates the need for memorization and calculation, which are major sources of error in pediatric weight estimation and drug dosage calculations.[2]

CLARK'S RULE

Clark's Rule is more accurate than Fried's Rule and Young's Rule. It may be applied to children over 2 years of age. It prorates a dose based on a ratio comparing the weight of the child to the weight of a standard adult.

$$\frac{\text{weight in pounds}}{150} * \text{adult dose} = \text{infant or child dose}$$

Exhibit 9-8 Clark's Rule

The child's weight, in pounds, is divided by 150 lb, which represents a standard adult weight. This calculates a ratio of body mass between the child and a standard adult. This ratio is then multiplied by the standard adult dose to calculate the child's dose.

FRIED'S RULE

Fried's Rule applies to infants under 1 year of age and is based on age in months.

$$\frac{\text{age in months}}{150} * \text{adult dose} = \text{infant dose}$$

Exhibit 9-9 Fried's Rule

The child's age in months is divided by the weight of a standard adult in pounds (150 lb). This ratio is then multiplied by the standard adult dose to calculate the infant dose.

---

[1] Seidel JS, Chameides L, Luten RC, Zaritsky AL, Campbell FW. (June 1988). A Rapid Method for Estimating Weight and Resuscitation Drug Dosages from Length in the Pediatric Age Group. *Annals of Emergency Medicine, 17*(6), 576/43–580/47.
[2] Ibid.

YOUNG'S RULE

Young's Rule, named after Thomas Young, is another rule based on age, but it applies to children under 12 years of age rather than infants. The child's age in years is divided by itself plus 12. This number is then multiplied by the standard adult dose to calculate the pediatric dose.

$$\frac{\text{age in years}}{\text{age} + 12} * \text{adult dose} = \text{child dose}$$

Exhibit 9-10 Young's Rule

The example in Exhibit 9-11 calculates a pediatric dose with each of the formulas for a medication with an adult dose of 100 mg. The child's age differs in the example of Fried's Rule because that rule applies only to children under the age of 1.

Clark's Rule

$$\frac{\text{weight in pounds}}{150} * \text{adult dose} = \text{infant or child dose}$$

$\frac{45}{150} * 100 \text{ mg} = \text{dose}$	Clark's Rule is applied to a 6-year-old, 45 lb child and a medicine with a standard adult dose of 100 mg.

30 mg = dose

Fried's Rule

$$\frac{\text{age in months}}{150} * \text{adult dose} = \text{infant dose}$$

$\frac{8}{150} * 100 \text{ mg} = \text{dose}$	Fried's Rule is applied to an 8-month-old infant and a medicine with a standard adult dose of 100 mg.

5.34 mg = dose

Young's Rule

$$\frac{\text{age in years}}{\text{age} + 12} * \text{adult dose} = \text{child dose}$$

$\frac{6}{6 + 12} * 100 \text{ mg} = \text{dose}$	Young's Rule is applied to a 6-year-old child and a medicine with a standard adult dose of 100 mg.

33.3 mg = dose

Exhibit 9-11 Comparative Pediatric Dosage Calculations

BODY SURFACE AREA

The skin is the largest human organ. Some medication dosages are based on the area of the skin. The area of the skin is the body surface area (BSA), sometimes referred to as "total body surface area."

The easiest method of determining the body surface area is to use one of the normal body surface area charts, such as the West Nomogram. This chart uses the patient's body measurements and plots a body surface area without requiring calculations.

WEST NOMOGRAM

To use the West Nomogram, draw a line from the adult patient's height on the left to the patient's weight on the right. The body surface area will be displayed on the scale marked "SA" (surface area) for adults. For pediatric patients, use the weight and surface area chart on the scale marked "For children of normal height for weight."

PEDIATRIC BSA RULE OF THUMB

A formula that may be used, in the absence of a nomogram or other tables, to approximate the body surface area in cubic meters of a child patient is shown in Exhibit 9-12. (The values there are rounded off to the number of significant digits.)

Formula: $\dfrac{(4 * \text{child's weight in kilograms}) + 7}{\text{child's weight in kilograms} + 90} = \text{BSA in square meters}$

Example: Calculate the approximate BSA for a 60.85 lb (27.66 kg) child

$\dfrac{(4 * 27.66) + 7}{27.66 + 90} = \text{BSA in square meters}$

$\dfrac{(110.64) + 7}{117.66} = \text{BSA in square meters}$

$\dfrac{117.7}{117.7} = \text{BSA in square meters}$

$1 \text{ m}^2 = \text{BSA}$

Exhibit 9-12 Pediatric Rule of Thumb for Body Surface Area

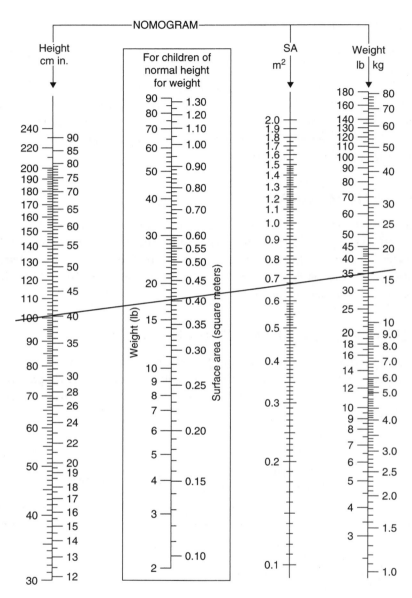

Pediatric doses of medications are generally based on body surface area (BSA) or weight. To calculate a child's BSA, draw a straight line from the height (in the left-hand column) to the weight (in the right-hand column). The point at which the line intersects the surface area (SA) column is the BSA (measured in square meters [m²]). If the child is of roughly normal proportion, BSA can be calculated from the weight alone (in the enclosed area).

Source: Vaughan VC, McKay RJ (eds.). (1983). *Nelson Textbook of Pediatrics,* 12th ed. Philadelphia: Saunders. Reprinted with permission.

Figure 9-5 West Nomogram

CONCENTRATION FORMULA

Some clinicians use a shortcut to the ratio equation method of determining a dose. This concentration formula (Exhibit 9-13) can be applied to concentration problems. It uses the ratio equation method but skips the first stage of the set-up and starts immediately at the second stage of factoring x.

The formula is derived in the following manner. It uses different terms than those that have been previously used in this text, but the set-up is the same. "Dose" represents the unknown. "Quantity" and "have" represent the volume and mass of concentration. And "Order" represents the information referenced to the unknown.

$$\frac{(d) \text{ dose}}{(o) \text{ order}} = \frac{(q) \text{ quantity}}{(h) \text{ have}}$$

The equation is solved to the second stage before substituting real values in the place of the unknowns. The formula actually represents the second stage of a routine ratio concentration equation.

$$(d) \text{ dose} = \frac{(q) \text{ quantity}}{(h) \text{ have}} * (o) \text{ order}$$

$$d = \frac{q}{h} * o \qquad \text{This is the derived formula using letters to represent the words above.}$$

Example: The order is for 65 mg of lidocaine.

Known: The medication is supplied in a prefilled syringe containing 100 mg/10 ml of a 1% solution.

Unknown: How many milliliters are given?

$$d = \frac{10 \text{ ml}}{100 \text{ mg}} * 65 \text{ mg} \qquad \text{Use the concentration formula.}$$

$$d = \frac{650 \text{ ml}}{100}$$

$$d = 6.5 \text{ ml}$$

Exhibit 9-13 Generic Concentration Dose Formula

The disadvantage of the concentration formula is, if the clinician does not understand the process for setting up equations, the clinician may be confused on determining whether to set up for volume or concentration.

HENDERSON–HASSELBALCH EQUATION

The Henderson–Hasselbalch equation (Exhibit 9-14) is the underlying principal used to calculate the pH (i.e., hydrogen ion) concentration of average blood serum. This equation is named for Lawrence Joseph Henderson

(1878–1942), an American chemist, and Karl A. Hasselbalch (1874–1962), a Copenhagen scientist.

$$pH = pK_a + log_{10} \frac{(A^-)}{(HA)}$$

$$pH = pK_a + log_{10} \frac{(HCO_3^-)}{PaCO_2 * (0.03 \text{ mEq/L/mmHg})}$$

A^- represents an acid (HCO_3^- measurement).

HA represents a weak acid in solution (the $PaCO_2$ measurement).

pK_a is the 6.1 (dissociation constant for carbonic acid).

$PaCO_2$ is 40. HCO_3^- is measured. The pH may be calculated if the measured HCO_3^- is known.

Exhibit 9-14 Henderson–Hasselbalch Equation

The serum pH is equal to the pK_a (6.1), plus the logarithm of HCO_3^- (the bicarbonate measurement), divided by the $PaCO_2$, times 0.03 mEq/L/mmHg (the partial arterial [Pa] measure of dissolved carbon dioxide) (Exhibit 9-15). Do not be alarmed if this is confusing. This is technical and is not directly useful for dosage calculations. It is the equation on which acid-base balance calculations (see Chapter 10) are based. The 0.03 mEq/L/mmHg is a unit conversion factor to convert the $PaCO_2$ from millimeters of mercury (Hg) to milliequivalents.

Formula: $pH = pK_a + log_{10} \dfrac{(HCO_3)}{PaCO_2 * (0.03 \text{ mEq/L/mmHg})}$

Example: Calculate the pH, given a $PaCO_2$ of 40 mmHg and a HCO_3^- of 24 mEq/L

$$pH = 6.10 + \frac{\log (24 \text{ mEq/L})}{40 \text{ mmHg} * (0.03 \text{ mEq/L/mmHg})}$$

$$pH = 6.10 + \frac{\log (24 \text{ mEq/L})}{1.2 \text{ mEq/L}}$$

$$pH = 6.10 + \log(20)$$

$$pH = 6.10 + 1.30 = 7.4$$

Exhibit 9-15 Calculation of Normal Midrange (7.35–7.45) pH

REVIEW PROBLEMS

An adult is burned on the front of both arms from the elbow to the hands. What is the percent of the burn?

1. Using the Rule of Nines _____

2. Using the Lund and Browder chart _____

An adult patient has a major burn with both full arms, the full anterior chest, and the full anterior abdomen burned. What is the percent of the burn?

3. Using the Rule of Nines _____

4. Using the Lund and Browder chart _____

A 14-month-old child is burned on the front of the upper torso and the tops of both arms. What is the percent of the burn?

5. Using the Rule of Nines _____

6. Using the Lund and Browder chart _____

7. Using the Parkland formula, what is the IV flow rate for a 180 lb patient with a 40% burn for the first 8 hours? _____

8. Using the Parkland formula, what is the IV flow rate for a 180 lb patient with a 40% burn for the 12th hour? _____

A 10-month-old child weighing 26.5 lb is prescribed a medication for which the normal adult dose is 50 mg. Calculate the dose using:

9. Clark's Rule _____

10. Fried's Rule _____

11. Young's Rule _____

Make the necessary conversions and complete this table:

Celsius	Fahrenheit
12. 37°C	_____ °F
13. _____ °C	101°F
14. _____ °C	0°F
15. 45°C	_____ °F
16. 32°C	_____ °F

Using the concentration formula, determine the following doses in milliliters given the concentration and order.

Concentration	Order	Volume
100 mg/10 ml	75 mg	17. _____
100 mg/5 ml	75 mg	18. _____
500 mg/10 ml	1 g	19. _____
1 mg/10 ml	0.5 mg	20. _____
1 mg/1 ml	0.3 mg	21. _____
0.5 mg/5 ml	1 mg	22. _____

23. Using the BSA rule of thumb, what is the BSA of a child who weighs 11 kg? _____

Using the Henderson-Hasselbalch equation, calculate:

24. The pH, given a $PaCO_2$ of 40 and an HCO_3^- of 38.4 mEq/L _____

25. The pH, given a $PaCO_2$ of 40 and an HCO_3^- of 22 mEq/L _____

Chapter 10

Acid-Base Balance

A failure is not always a mistake; it may simply be the best one can do under the circumstances.

The real mistake is to stop trying.

—B. F. Skinner, *Beyond Freedom and Dignity.*

Exhibit 10-1

OBJECTIVES

Upon completion of this chapter the clinician should be able to:

1. Recognize upscale and downscale changes on a numerical scale that uses both positive and negative numbers
2. Perform addition and subtraction of negative numbers
3. Determine the absolute value of negative numbers
4. Use unit conversion factors to convert between pH, Torr, and milliequivalent units of measure
5. Use a unit conversion factor to convert between weight in pounds and weight in kilograms
6. Solve equations using the correct order of operations

KEY TERMS

acidosis	correct
alkalosis	exponent
balance	extracellular fluid
base	golden rules
carbonic acid	log
compensate	logarithm

negative log   relative base deficit
Pa   Torr
pH

INTRODUCTION TO ACID-BASE BALANCE

The human body maintains homeostasis of temperature and chemical balance. This homeostasis is a complex biochemical process that involves multiple processes and feedback loops. Acid-base balance is one of the homeostatic processes that the body maintains. The acid-base level is measured in **pH**, which is the reciprocal **logarithm** of the concentration of hydrogen ions in solution in the blood. As the pH value becomes larger, the concentration of hydrogen ions becomes smaller and vice versa. The more hydrogen ions present, the more the blood is acidic. Therefore, as the pH gets smaller, the hydrogen ion concentration gets larger and the blood becomes more acidic.

The human body requires an acid-base balance in the pH range of 7.36 to 7.44. Deviations below 7.36 are considered acidotic, and those above 7.44 are alkalotic. **Acidosis** and **alkalosis** are opposite problems in maintaining acid-base **balance**. Acidosis is too much acid. Alkalosis is too little acid.

Abnormalities in pH balance create serious repercussions in overall homeostasis. The hemoglobin in the blood is unable to normally transport oxygen. Other electrolytes (ions) in the blood are imbalanced. Electrolyte imbalance may create disturbances in cardiac rhythm. The effects of medications are usually impaired in either an acidotic or alkalotic condition.

It is important to carefully **compensate** or **correct** for significant acid-base imbalance with medication. This correction should be guided by blood tests called *arterial blood gas* (*ABGs*) *tests*. If too much medication is given, the imbalance is overcorrected, creating the opposite problem and the clinician has violated the basic rule of "do no harm."

ACID-BASE CALCULATIONS

Acid-base balance concepts and calculations are not difficult. The arterial blood gas measurements are made in pH and **Torr**. The medication is administered in milliequivalents (mEq). These units require unit conversion factors to calculate the required dose. There are several steps to remember.

However, if the calculations are approached one step at a time, they may be reduced to simple mathematical operations of conversion of units of Torr to units of pH, subtraction of like terms (units of pH), conversion of units of pH to units of milliequivalents, multiplication, and division.

The American Heart Association (AHA) no longer requires calculation of bicarbonate dosages for patients with acid-base imbalance. This material is optional for allied health professionals. The AHA established three **golden rules** that are unit conversion factors by which arterial blood measurements may be converted to like terms.[1] Arterial blood gases are measured in Torr and pH. Bicarbonate dosages are measured in milliequivalents. The golden rules allow conversions between Torr, pH, and milliequivalents (Exhibit 10-2). These constants are just like the known constants of 60 min/hr or 2.2 lb/kg.

Golden rule 1 is a unit conversion factor to convert between units of pH and Torr:

$$+10 \text{ Torr}: -0.08 \text{ pH}$$

Golden Rule 2 is a unit conversion factor to convert between units of pH and milliequivalents:

$$-0.15 \text{ pH}:10 \text{ mEq}$$

Golden Rule 3 gives a guideline for calculating liters of extracellular fluid (ECF) based on patient weight:

$$\text{dose} = \frac{\text{(base deficit/liters of ECF) (patient weight in kilograms)}}{4}$$

Source: McIntyre KM, Lewis AJ, Carveth SW (eds.). (1983). *Textbook of Advanced Cardiac Life Support,* 1st ed. Dallas, TX: American Heart Association.

Exhibit 10-2 The Golden Rules of Acid-Base Balance

Arterial blood gas measurements analyze blood for content of carbon dioxide and pH. The acidity of the body is determined by a balance of carbon dioxide (which forms an acid when dissolved in blood) and metabolic acid level.

Excess carbon dioxide is treated by ventilation. Metabolic acids are treated by intravenous administration of bicarbonate. The dosage of bicarbonate is guided by calculating the amount of metabolic acid that is present.

The ABG measurement does not directly reflect metabolic acidosis. It shows the total blood acid level, which includes the respiratory acid level and metabolic acid level. The clinician can figure the metabolic acid level by

---

[1] McIntyre KM, Lewis AJ, Carveth SW (eds.). (1983). *Textbook of Advanced Cardiac Life Support,* 1st ed. Dallas, TX: American Heart Association.

taking the pH of the blood and subtracting the respiratory component (Exhibit 10-3). The respiratory and metabolic components use different units of measure; therefore, before subtraction, unit conversion factors must be used to convert them to into similar units.

---

total acid level (measured in pH) = respiratory acid (measured in Torr) + metabolic acid

metabolic acid = total acid level (in pH) − respiratory acid (in Torr)

The metabolic component must be calculated by subtracting the respiratory component of acid levels from the total acid levels. The measurements for the respiratory and total acid levels are in different units (Torr or pH), so a unit conversion factor converts them to a common form. The golden rules provide unit conversion factors for this calculation.

It is important to note metabolic or respiratory changes in acid level may be to a higher-than-normal or to a lower-than-normal measurement. Positive or negative signs are very important, signaling the clinician to treat acidosis or alkalosis.

The average values of arterial blood gases is a pH of 7.4 and a $PaCO_2$ of 40 Torr.

Exhibit 10-3 Calculating the Metabolic Component

Blood is **extracellular fluid** (ECF). The theory is that acidosis or alkalosis may be treated by treating the blood, which is extracellular fluid. The amount of ECF also must be calculated. The treatment is based on liters of ECF. Liters of ECF may be approximately calculated by dividing the patient's body weight in kilograms by 4. The pH and $PaCO_2$ are the only two measurements required to calculate acid-base balance and the dose of sodium bicarbonate to correct metabolic acidosis. These measurements are in different units and must be converted to common units using unit conversion factors.

Respiratory and metabolic acidosis are managed differently. Respiratory acid-base imbalance problems are managed with ventilation. Only metabolic acidosis is managed with an IV bolus of sodium bicarbonate. The equation to calculate the dose is found in Exhibit 10-4.

---

dose = metabolic acidosis ∗ liters of ECF

dose = (measured pH change − respiratory pH change) ∗ (liters of ECF)

Exhibit 10-4 Bicarbonate Dosage Formula

Metabolic acidosis is caused by any condition that generates excess metabolic acids in the system. The most common cause is excessive lactic acid from anaerobic metabolism that occurs when the patient is in respiratory or cardiac arrest. Medical conditions such as diabetes may also cause metabolic acidosis. Metabolic alkalosis occurs when metabolic acids are removed from the body, which happens during acute diarrhea or acute vomiting. Metabolic alkalosis may also be caused by administering too much metabolic **base** when treating metabolic acidosis. Treatment of metabolic acidosis should always be guided by arterial blood gas measurements. Remember the primary admonition to health care providers of "first, do no harm." A clinician cannot remove bicarbonate once it has been administered. Treat metabolic acidosis most carefully to ensure you do not convert it to metabolic alkalosis.

The bicarbonate dose, pH, and respiratory pH are all measured in different units: milliequivalents, pH, and Torr. These must, as mentioned before, be converted to like units, using unit conversion factors. The liters of ECF are also calculated using the guideline that ECF is equal to one fourth the patient's body weight in kilograms.

Acid base balancing and the calculation of a sodium bicarbonate dose, if necessary, requires 2 unit conversions: a simple subtraction and division by 4. The use of unit conversion factors between these units and the need for several steps can be confusing. Exhibit 10-5 shows the four steps of subtraction, the two unit conversions, and the division. The use of these steps can simplify what may first appear mystifying.

The clinician does not need to proceed beyond the subtraction step if subtraction indicates that the acidosis is all respiratory and that no base deficit exists. This is because a sodium bicarbonate dose is not needed. Remember, sodium bicarbonate is only given for metabolic acidosis and is not normally given for respiratory acidosis.

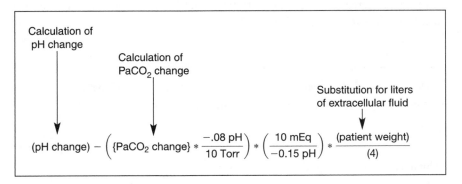

Exhibit 10-5 Putting the Formulas Together

THE pH MEASUREMENT

As previously explained, *pH* stands for the scale of hydrogen ions in the solution being measured. Hydrogen ions are acid ions, so by measuring the concentration of hydrogen ions in solution, the concentration of acid is directly measured.

A logarithm uses scientific notation. Scientific notation is a shorthand system used to express very large or very small numbers by writing the number as a power of 10. For example, 1 times 10^9 is 10 raised to the 9th power, or 1 billion. A logarithm is the **exponent** of 10 that is used in scientific notation. For example, the **log** 2 represents 1 times 10^2, or 100. The log 4 represents 1 times 10 raised to the 4th power, which is 10,000. A log of 3.25 represents a number larger than 1 times 10^3 (1,000) and a smaller one than 1 times 10 to the 4th power (10,000). The number can be found in a logarithm table (as shown in Exhibit 10-6) or calculated.

Number	100	1,000	10,000	100,000
Scientific notation	$1 * 10^2$	$1 * 10^3$	$1 * 10^4$	$1 * 10^5$
Log	2	3	4	5

Exhibit 10-6 Sample Logarithmic Scale

A negative logarithm scale measures a fraction. It represents 1 divided by the value of the logarithm. Expressed another way, a negative logarithm is the reciprocal of a positive logarithm. As a negative log increases, the denominator increases. As the denominator increases, the value of the fraction decreases, as shown in Exhibit 10-7.

Number	0.01	0.001	0.0001	0.00001
Scientific notation	$1 * 10^{-2}$	$1 * 10^{-3}$	$1 * 10^{-4}$	$1 * 10^{-5}$
Log	−2	−3	−4	−5

Exhibit 10-7 Sample Negative Logarithmic Scale

The pH scale measures concentrations on a negative logarithm scale from 1 to 14. The negative sign is not used because, by definition, the pH scale is a **negative log** (concentration) scale. As the negative log on the pH scale increases, the concentration of hydrogen ions decreases and the solution becomes less acidic. For example, a value of 8 is 10 times less acidic than a value of 7.

THE PaCO$_2$ MEASUREMENT

The **Pa** designation in PaCO$_2$ stands for the *partial arterial pressure* of the gas carbon dioxide. Carbon dioxide is dissolved in the blood. Gases are measured in millimeters of mercury (mmHg) like blood pressure. The term *Torr* is used as a unit of measure of millimeters of mercury when discussing gas pressure in solution.

There are several gases dissolved in arterial blood. The most significant two are carbon dioxide and oxygen. Only carbon dioxide and pH measurements are required to calculate dosages for the neutralization of metabolic acidosis. Carbon dioxide dissolves under pressure in blood serum by combining with water to form **carbonic acid** (H$_2$CO$_3$). Carbon dioxide in solution contributes to the body's acidosis by combining with fluid to form carbonic acid. The normal amount of carbon dioxide is 40 mmHg, or 40 Torr. This is the pressure required to raise mercury 40 mm in a vertical tube. A measurement of more than 40 Torr represents too much carbonic acid, which is respiratory acidosis. A measurement less than 40 Torr represents too little carbonic acid, which is respiratory alkalosis.

Respiratory acidosis may be caused by any disease or injury that decreases respiratory effort. These include pneumonia, fractured ribs with pain-inhibited respiration, congestive heart failure with pulmonary edema, etc. Respiratory alkalosis results from excessive ventilation—voiding too much carbon dioxide—which in turn causes carbonic acid to shift to water and carbon dioxide. This could result from hyperventilation induced by excessive ventilation by health care providers, hysteria, a head injury, or a drug overdose.

To calculate the respiratory change, subtract 40 Torr from the measured PaCO$_2$. If the result is a positive number, it represents respiratory acidosis. If the number is negative, it represents respiratory alkalosis. For some examples, see Exhibit 10-8.

Respiratory value

75 Torr	
70 Torr	
65 Torr	
60 Torr	
55 Torr	
50 Torr	
45 Torr	Acidosis
40 Torr	Average balance
35 Torr	Alkalosis
30 Torr	
25 Torr	
20 Torr	
15 Torr	
10 Torr	
5 Torr	

Example of a metabolic acidotic measurement:

$PaCO_2$: 50 Torr

50 Torr − 40 Torr = +10 Torr: (respiratory acidosis)

Example of a metabolic alkalotic measurement:

$PaCO_2$: 35 Torr

35 Torr − 40 Torr = −5 Torr: (respiratory alkalosis)

Exhibit 10-8 Respiratory Acid Balance

Exhibit 10-9 is a short exercise in assessing respiratory acid balance.

Measured $PaCO_2$	Acidosis or alkalosis	Torr change
25 Torr	_____	_____
30 Torr	_____	_____
35 Torr	alkalosis	−5 Torr
45 Torr	_____	_____
50 Torr	acidosis	+10 Torr
55 Torr	_____	_____

Exhibit 10-9 Respiratory Analysis Exercise

The American Heart Association's Golden Rule 1 (Exhibit 10-10) provides a unit conversion factor to convert Torr of respiratory acid to pH. That ratio is $+10$ Torr -0.08 pH change. An increase in respiratory acid is associated with a downscale (or decrease) in pH.

+10 Torr : −0.08 pH

To convert a measured $PaCO_2$ to pH, use this ratio as a unit conversion factor.

$$\frac{15 \text{ torr } (-0.08 \text{ pH})}{+10 \text{ torr}} = 0.12 \text{ pH (respiratory component of the pH change)}$$

Source: McIntyre KM, Lewis AJ, Carveth SW (eds.). (1983). *Textbook of Advanced Cardiac Life Support,* 1st ed. Dallas, TX: American Heart Association.

Exhibit 10-10 Golden Rule 1

If there is excess respiratory acid, the patient has respiratory acidosis. The pH change will be downscale (or negative). If there is deficit respiratory acid, the patient has respiratory alkalosis. The pH change will be upscale (or positive). Exhibit 10-11 is a short exercise in determining respiratory acid balance and pH.

Measured $PaCO_2$	Acidosis or alkalosis	Torr change	pH factor
25 Torr	_____	_____	_____
30 Torr	_____	_____	_____
35 Torr	alkalosis	−5 Torr	+0.04 pH
45 Torr	_____	_____	_____
50 Torr	acidosis	+10 Torr	−0.08 pH
55 Torr	_____	_____	_____

Exhibit 10-11 Respiratory pH Analysis Exercise

Respiratory acidosis, which is an excess of carbon dioxide, is normally managed by increasing ventilation to cause carbon dioxide to be breathed off. Respiratory alkalosis, which is a deficit of carbon dioxide, is managed by decreasing (when safe) ventilation, which causes carbon dioxide to be retained.

METABOLIC ANALYSIS

Metabolic acidosis results from the generation of excess acid or a deficit of base. Metabolic acid levels cannot be measured directly. The only way to measure acid levels is by an arterial pH analysis, which measures the body's total acid-base balance. This includes both respiratory acid and the metabolic acids and bases. To determine what the metabolic acidosis is, the clinician can subtract the respiratory part from the total pH. The respiratory acid is measured in Torr, while total acid-base balance is measured in pH. The respiratory acid must be converted from a Torr measurement to a pH measurement before subtraction.

The American Heart Association's Golden Rule 1 provides a unit conversion factor to convert Torr of carbon dioxide to pH. A pH of 7.4 represents the average of acceptable pH ranges (7.36–7.44 pH) in the human body. The pH change (from normal) is the measured pH minus the normal pH. If the answer is negative, there is a downscale pH change, which represents acidosis, as shown in Exhibit 10-12.

A measured pH of 7.3 indicates a downscale change, so we expect this to represent acidosis. The mathematical equation verifies our expectation.

measured pH − average pH = pH change

7.3 pH   − 7.4 pH   = −0.1 pH

The pH change is −0.1. The negative value indicates an acidotic change.

Exhibit 10-12 pH Analysis

If the pH change is equal to zero, then there is no measurable pH change, and the blood's acid-base levels are either balanced or compensated. If the pH change is within ±0.04 pH, then the measured pH is within normal limits (7.36–7.44 pH). If the pH change is less than –0.04 (such as –0.05 pH), there is a downscale change, which indicates acidosis. If the pH change is more positive than +0.04 (such as +0.05), there is an upscale change, which indicates alkalosis. Exhibit 10-13 is a short exercise in determining respiratory pH change.

Measured pH	Alkalosis or acidosis	Average pH	pH change
7.3 pH	acidosis	7.4 pH	−0.1 pH
7.4 pH	_____	7.4 pH	_____
7.5 pH	_____	7.4 pH	_____
7.32 pH	_____	7.4 pH	_____
7.25 pH	_____	7.4 pH	_____
7.55 pH	_____	7.4 pH	_____
7.38 pH	_____	7.4 pH	_____

Exhibit 10-13 pH Change Exercise

If the pH change indicates acidosis, the clinician must determine how much of the acidosis is metabolic and how much is respiratory. This distinction must be made because the two types of acidosis are managed differently. Respiratory acidosis is managed with ventilation. Metabolic acidosis is managed with both sodium bicarbonate and ventilation. Administration of sodium bicarbonate causes a generation of additional CO_2, which must be ventilated. It is imperative not to neglect ventilation in managing metabolic acidosis. Exhibit 10-14 is an exercise in determining acid-base balance based on both the pH and the measured Torr.

Measured pH factor	Measured PaCO$_2$	Measured Torr change	Metabolic pH change	Measured pH change	Respiratory pH change
7.30	ex. −0.10	40 Torr	−0 pH	−0.10	−0.10
7.32	40 Torr	_____	_____	_____	_____
7.25	40 Torr	_____	_____	_____	_____
7.15	40 Torr	_____	_____	_____	_____
7.20	40 Torr	_____	_____	_____	_____
7.30	50 Torr	_____	_____	_____	_____
7.32	50 Torr	_____	_____	_____	_____
7.25	50 Torr	_____	_____	_____	_____
7.15	50 Torr	_____	_____	_____	_____
7.20	50 Torr	_____	_____	_____	_____
7.40	50 Torr	_____	_____	_____	_____
7.40	30 Torr	_____	_____	_____	_____
7.30	30 Torr	_____	_____	_____	_____
7.32	30 Torr	_____	_____	_____	_____
7.25	30 Torr	_____	_____	_____	_____
7.15	30 Torr	_____	_____	_____	_____
7.20	30 Torr	_____	_____	_____	_____

Exhibit 10-14 Acid-Base Balance Exercise

If the metabolic pH change is zero, the patient has no metabolic acid-base imbalance. If the metabolic pH change is positive, the patient has metabolic alkalosis. If the metabolic pH change is negative, the patient has metabolic acidosis. A sodium bicarbonate dosage should be calculated based on the patient's weight.

DETERMINATION OF DOSAGE

Metabolic acidosis has been calculated in units of pH. It is also called the **relative base deficit** because it is a measure of the absolute value of base that must be given to neutralize the acidosis. A milliequivalent is the metric unit of measure for electrolyte medications, rather than pH or milligrams. The sodium bicarbonate dosage is expressed in milliequivalents because it is an electrolyte medication. A unit conversion factor is used to convert the absolute value of the metabolic deficit to milliequivalents.

The American Heart Association's Golden Rule 2 provides a unit conversion factor to convert units of pH to milliequivalents (Exhibit 10-15). That ratio is –0.15 pH change is equal to +10 mEq.

-0.15 pH:10 mEq

Source: McIntyre KM, Lewis AJ, Carveth SW (eds.). (1983). *Textbook of Advanced Cardiac Life Support,* 1st ed. Dallas, TX: American Heart Association.

Exhibit 10-15 Golden Rule 2

Arterial blood gas measurements are measured in units per liter of ECF. The last step in determining the total dose is to multiply the dose by the number of liters of ECF. Golden Rule 3 gives a unit conversion factor to convert from the patient's weight in kilograms to liters of ECF, as shown in Exhibit 10-16.

$$\text{dose} = \frac{(\text{base deficit})\ (\text{patient weight in kilograms})}{4}$$

Source: McIntyre KM, Lewis AJ, Carveth SW (eds.). (1983). *Textbook of Advanced Cardiac Life Support,* 1st ed. Dallas, TX: American Heart Association.

Exhibit 10-16 Golden Rule 3

The number of liters of ECF may be calculated. The American Heart Association guideline states that ECF accounts for one quarter of the body's total weight. A liter of water is equal to a kilogram. The number of liters of the patient's body fluids is approximately equal to the patient's weight in kg. One quarter of the patient's fluid is extracellular.

The liters of extracellular fluid then are equal to one quarter the total body weight (in kilograms).

REVIEW OF CALCULATION STEPS

The steps to dosage determination, given the $PaCO_2$ in Torr and the pH of arterial blood, are:

1. Calculate the pH change from normal pH (using the average pH of 7.4).
2. Calculate the $PaCO_2$ change from normal $PaCO_2$ (using the average of 40 Torr).
3. If metabolic acidosis is present, determine the dosage by multiplying those milliequivalents by one fourth the patient's body weight in kilograms.

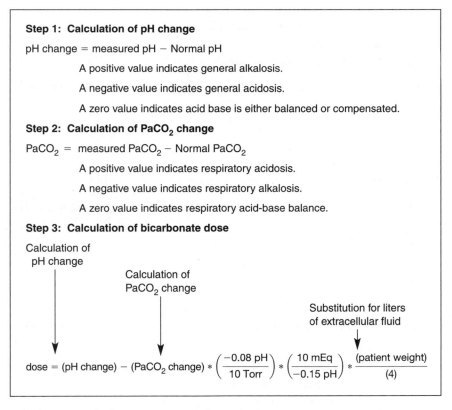

Step 1: Calculation of pH change

pH change = measured pH − Normal pH

       A positive value indicates general alkalosis.

       A negative value indicates general acidosis.

       A zero value indicates acid base is either balanced or compensated.

Step 2: Calculation of $PaCO_2$ change

$PaCO_2$ = measured $PaCO_2$ − Normal $PaCO_2$

       A positive value indicates respiratory acidosis.

       A negative value indicates respiratory alkalosis.

       A zero value indicates respiratory acid-base balance.

Step 3: Calculation of bicarbonate dose

Calculation of pH change

Calculation of $PaCO_2$ change

Substitution for liters of extracellular fluid

$$\text{dose} = (\text{pH change}) - (PaCO_2 \text{ change}) * \left(\frac{-0.08 \text{ pH}}{10 \text{ Torr}}\right) * \left(\frac{10 \text{ mEq}}{-0.15 \text{ pH}}\right) * \frac{(\text{patient weight})}{(4)}$$

Exhibit 10-17 Bicarbonate Dose Template Equation

> We shall not cease from exploration
> And the end of all our exploring
> Will be to arrive where we started
> And know the place for the first time.
>
> —T. S. Eliot.

Exhibit 10-18

REVIEW PROBLEMS

A patient has a $PaCO_2$ of 40 Torr and a pH of 7.30. The patient's weight is 110 lb.

1. The patient's pH change is _____.
2. The patient's respiratory pH factor is _____.
3. The patient's metabolic pH factor is _____.
4. The patient's base deficit is _____ mEq/L.
5. The correct sodium bicarbonate dosage is _____ mEq.

A patient has a $PaCO_2$ of 50 Torr and a pH of 7.22. The patient's weight is 110 lb.

6. The patient's pH change is _____.
7. The patient's respiratory pH factor is _____.
8. The patient's metabolic pH factor is _____.
9. The patient's base deficit is _____ mEq/L.
10. The correct sodium bicarbonate dosage is _____ mEq.

A patient has a $PaCO_2$ of 30 Torr and a pH of 7.30. The patient's weight is 110 lb.

11. The patient's pH change is _____.
12. The patient's respiratory pH factor is _____.
13. The patient's metabolic pH factor is _____.
14. The patient's base deficit is _____ mEq/L.
15. The correct sodium bicarbonate dosage is _____ mEq.

A patient has a $PaCO_2$ of 40 Torr and a pH of 7.17. The patient's weight is 110 lb.

16. The patient's pH change is _____.
17. The patient's respiratory pH factor is _____.
18. The patient's metabolic pH factor is _____.
19. The patient's base deficit is _____ mEq/L.
20. The correct sodium bicarbonate dosage is _____ mEq.

A patient has a $PaCO_2$ of 60 Torr and a pH of 7.14. The patient's weight is 185 lb.

21. The patient's pH change is _____.
22. The patient's respiratory pH factor is _____.
23. The patient's metabolic pH factor is _____.
24. The patient's base deficit is _____ mEq/L.
25. The correct sodium bicarbonate dosage is _____ mEq.

A patient has a $PaCO_2$ of 45 Torr and a pH of 7.31. The patient's weight is 132 lb.

26. The patient's pH change is _____.
27. The patient's respiratory pH factor is _____.
28. The patient's metabolic pH factor is _____.
29. The patient's base deficit is _____ mEq/L.
30. The correct sodium bicarbonate dosage is _____ mEq.

A patient has a $PaCO_2$ of 35 Torr and a pH of 7.44. The patient's weight is 165 lb.

31. The patient's pH change is _____.
32. The patient's respiratory pH factor is _____.
33. The patient's metabolic pH factor is _____.
34. The patient's base deficit is _____ mEq/L.
35. The correct sodium bicarbonate dosage is _____ mEq.

A patient has a $PaCO_2$ of 40 Torr and a pH of 7.10. The patient's weight is 165 lb.

36. The patient's pH change is _____.
37. The patient's respiratory pH factor is _____.
38. The patient's metabolic pH factor is _____.
39. The patient's base deficit is _____ mEq/L.
40. The correct sodium bicarbonate dosage is _____ mEq.

A patient has a $PaCO_2$ of 70 Torr and a pH of 7.40. The patient's weight is 220 lb.

41. The patient's pH change is _____.
42. The patient's respiratory pH factor is _____.
43. The patient's metabolic pH factor is _____.
44. The patient's base deficit is _____ mEq/L.
45. The correct sodium bicarbonate dosage is _____ mEq.

A patient has a PaCO$_2$ of 70 Torr and a pH of 7.40. The patient's weight is 88 lb.

46. The patient's pH change is _____.
47. The patient's respiratory pH factor is _____.
48. The patient's metabolic pH factor is _____.
49. The patient's base deficit is _____ mEq/L.
50. The correct sodium bicarbonate dosage is _____ mEq.

Review Problems: Answer Key

That's what learning is, after all; not whether we lose the game, but how we lose and how we've changed because of it and what we take away from it that we never had before, to apply to other games. Losing, in a curious way, is winning.

—Richard Bach, *Bridge Across Forever.*

CHAPTER 2

1. 15
2. 15
3. 15
4. 15
5. 20
6. 10
7. 4
8. 6
9. 8
10. 1
11. 1.5
12. 2
13. 16
14. 1
15. 0.44
16. 4 quarters
17. 1 quarter
18. 4 qt
19. 2 qt
20. 2 qt
21. 1 qt
22. 0.5 case
23. 0.5 case
24. 16 ml
25. 2 ml
26. 15 mg/ml
27. 15 ml/mg
28. 0.25 mg/ml
29. 0.25 ml/mg
30. 1 mg
31. 1 ml
32. 1 ml
33. 5 mg
34. 5 mg
35. 20 mg
36. 10 mcg
37. 20 g
38. 10 mg
39. 5 g
40. 25 g
41. 0.2 g
42. 1 g
43. 1 g
44. 4 g
45. 1 g
46. 4 g
47. 1 g
48. 4 g
49. 1 L
50. 4 L

CHAPTER 3

1. 3,500; 0.0035; 0.035
2. 35,000; 0.035; 0.35
3. 350,000; 0.35; 3.5
4. 1000; 0.001; 0.01
5. 250; 0.00025; 0.0025
6. 50,000 mg; 0.05 mg; 0.5 mg
7. 1,354,000; 1.354; 13.54
8. 1/1,000; 0.001
9. 1/1,000,000; 0.000001
10. 1/1,000,000,000; 0.000000001
11. 10; 10
12. 100; 100
13. 1,000; 1,000
14. meter
15. gram
16. liter
17. International System of Units
18. 2.2 lb/1 kg
19. 1 kg/1,000 g
20. 1 g/1,000 mg
21. 1,000 g/1 kg
22. 1,000 mg/1 g
23. 1,000,000 ng/1 mg
24. 1,000 ml/1 L
25. 1 L/1,000 ml
26. 1 ml/1 g
27. 1,000 mm/1 m
28. 1 m/1,000 mm
29. 100 cm/1 m
30. 1 m/100 cm
31. 1 in/2.54 cm
32. 2.54 cm/1 in
33. 1 oz/30 ml
34. 30 ml/1 oz
35. 15.4 gr/1 g
36. 1 g/15.4 gr
37. 1 gr/64 mg
38. 1 mg/1,000,000 ng
39. 64 mg/1 gr
40. 1 km/1,000 m
41. 1,000 m/1 km
42. 1,000,000 mcg/1 g
43. 1 g/1,000,000 mcg
44. 1,000,000 ng/1 mg
45. 1 mcg/1,000 ng
46. 100 kg; 100,000,000 mg
47. 500 ml; 5 dcl
48. 5,000 ml; 0.5 dl
49. 250,000 mg; 250,000,000 mcg
50. 0.25 g; 250,000 mcg
51. 0.25 mg; 250,000 ng
52. 0.25 L; 250 g (of sterile water)
53. 0.64 g; 640 mg
54. 90 ml; 0.09 L
55. 0.06 L; 2 oz
56. 184.8 lb; 84,000,000 mg
57. 220,000,000 mg; 484 lb

[*Note:* For problems 58–72, metric conversions were not directly required but have been completed here to indicate a method of comparison.]

58. 5 cm (0.05 m)
59. 5 in (0.127 m)
60. 50 cm (0.5 in)
61. 1 yd (0.92 m)
62. 1 m (1.094 yd)
63. 500 ml
64. 1 qt (946 ml)
65. 1 L (1,000 ml)
66. 1 gal (3,784 ml)
67. 5,000 ml
68. 55,000 mg (0.055 kg)
69. 4,900 g (4.9 kg)
70. 100 lb (45 kg)
71. 49 kg
72. 55,000 (55 kg)

73. 0.454 kg; 454,000 mg
74. 50 kg; 50,000,000 mg
75. 84 kg; 84,000,000 mg
76. 165 lb; 75,000,000 mg
77. 211.8 kg; 211,800,000 mg
78. 454 g; 7,000 gr
79. 28.3 g; 28,300 mg
80. 30 ml; 30 g (of sterile water)
81. 15.4 gr
82. 64 mg
83. The metric system is a measurement system; the Arabic system is a numbering system.
84. A UCF is a ratio of two different units of measure that is equal to the whole number 1.
85. The metric system is more precise.
86. 1.3 gal
87. Approximately 20 t
88. 3.33 oz
89. 0.92 m
90. 0.353 oz
91. 946 ml
92. 30 ml
93. 3.84 L
94. 15.4 gr
95. 28.3 g
96. Approximately 5 ml
97. 64 mg
98. 0.3 m
99. 2.54 cm
100. 0.92 m

CHAPTER 4

1. 1 g
2. 0.001 ml
3. 1 g
4. 0.5 mg
5. 50 mg
6. 22 mg
7. 2.5 g
8. 22 mg
9. 1 mcg
10. 0.5 mg
11. 0.25 ml
12. 1,000 ml or 1 L
13. 0.25 ml
14. 1,000 ml or 1 L
15. 100 ml
16. 4 tablets
17. 100 ml
18. 4 tablets
19. 0.5 ml
20. 5 ml
21. 0.5 ml
22. 5 ml
23. 1,800 gtt
24. 2 ml
25. 1,800 gtt
26. 2 ml
27. 9 ml
28. 111 mg
29. 9 ml
30. 111 mg
31. 15 ml
32. 1,800 gtt
33. 15 ml
34. 220 ml
35. 1 ml
36. 1 ml
37. 0.2 mg
38. 0.2 mg

39. 0.2 mg
40. 12 tablets
41. 1 significant digit
42. 4 significant digits
43. 1 significant digit
44. 4 significant digits
45. 1 significant digit
46. 1 significant digit
47. 1 significant digit
48. millimeters and kilometers
49. grams and micrograms
50. meters and centimeters

CHAPTER 5

1. 1 mg/ml; 500 mg/500 ml
2. 2 mg/ml; 1 g/500 ml
3. 1 mcg/ml; 500 mg/500 ml
4. 1 ng/ml; 0.25 mg/250 ml
5. 2 mcg/ml; 0.5 mcg/250 ml
6. 4 mg/L; 4 mcg/ml
7. 1 g/250 ml; 4 mg/ml
8. 4 g/L; 1 g/250 ml
9. 4 mg/L; 1 mg/250 ml
10. 1,000 mcg/250 ml;
    4,000 mcg/L

11. 0.005 g
12. 100 mg
13. 250 ml
14. 2,500 ml
15. 700 mg
16. 50 kg
17. 5 ml
18. 0.5 ml
19. 3 g
20. 1 g
21. 1,000 mg (1 g)
22. 10 mg
23. 1,000 mg (1 g)
24. 10 ml
25. 3 g
26. 1.5 ml
27. 4 ml
28. 100 ml
29. 125 mg
30. 6.25 ml
31. 0.015 ml
32. 1.25 syringes
33. 2.5 ml
34. 500 mg
35. 5 ml
36. 4 units
37. 4 doses
38. 16 total daily units
39. 300 mg
40. 3 ml
41. 2 g (or 2,000 mg)
42. 2 syringes
43. 27.2 mEq
44. 84 mg
45. 8.4 ml
46. Parallelism involves placing like terms in the denominator while the term that is most like the unknown factor in the numerator.

47. Concentration is a given mass per unit of volume of a medication.
48. First, determine what is known.
49. Second, determine what is desired.
50. Third, set up an equation to solve for what is desired.

CHAPTER 6

1. 4 ml
2. 42.5 mg
3. 2.125 ml
4. 62.5 ml
5. 10 ml
6. 4 g
7. 25%
8. 0.25
9. 333%
10. 3.33
11. $\frac{1}{2}$
12. 0.5
13. $\frac{2}{3}$
14. 67%
15. 86.7%
16. 0.867
17. 167%
18. 1.67
19. 60%
20. 0.6
21. 16.6%
22. 0.167
23. 9/10
24. 0.9
25. $1\frac{3}{4}$
26. 1.75
27. $2\frac{1}{2}$
28. 2.5
29. 6
30. 6
31. 0.75
32. 0.75
33. 8
34. 8
35. 0
36. 0
37. 6.5 ml
38. 65 mg
39. yes
40. 3.25 ml
41. 0700
42. 1900
43. 1000
44. 2200
45. 2400 or 0000
46. 1200
47. 0.75 ml
48. Reconstitution is the process of adding a solvent to a powdered medication to reconstitute it to a fluid form.
49. Concentration is always found on the label of the medication as well as on its container.
50. Absolute value is the positive value of a number regardless of its arithmetic sign.

CHAPTER 7

1. 70 ml
2. 50%
3. 50 mEq
4. 50 mL
5. 1 mEq/ml
6. 50%
7. None
8. 50 mL
9. 50 mEq
10. 100 mL
11. 1 mEq/2 ml (or 0.5 mEq/ml)
12. 5 ml

13. 10%

14. 1 mg

15. 1 ml

16. 1 mg/ml

17. 90%

18. none

19. 9 ml

20. 1 mg

21. 10 ml

22. 1 mg/10 ml (or 0.1 mg/mL)

23. 200 mg

24. 4.25 ml

25. 10 ml

26. 50%

27. 1 g

28. 10 ml

29. 1 g/10 ml (or 100 mg/mL)

30. 50%

31. None

32. 10 ml

33. 1 g

34. 20 ml

35. 1 g/20 ml (or 50 mg/mL)

36. 50 ml

37. 1.5 ml

38. 6.7%

39. 15 mg

40. 1 ml

41. 15 mg/ml

42. 93.3%

43. None

44. 14 ml

45. 5 mg

46. 15 ml

47. 1 mg/ml

48. 7.5 mg

49. None; this is a 10% solution.

50. Titration is the concentration of a chemical solution that is sometimes manipulated to yield a specific effect.

CHAPTER 8

1. 4 mg/ml

2. 1 g/250 ml

3. 0.5 ml/min

4. 30 gtt/min

5. 2 mcg/ml

6. 1 mg/500 ml

7. 2 ml/min

8. 120 gtt/min

9. 8 mg/ml

10. 4 g/500 ml

11. 0.5 ml/min

12. 30 gtt/min

13. 4 mcg/ml

14. 1 mg/250 ml

15. 1.5 ml/min

16. 90 gtt/min

17. 8 mg/ml

18. 8 m/500 ml

19. 0.5 ml/min

20. 30 gtt/min

21. 2 mg/ml

22. 200 mg/100 ml

23. 0.5 ml/min

24. 30 gtt/min

25. 10 mg/ml

26. 5 g/500 ml

27. 0.5 ml/min

28. 30 gtt/min

29. 250 ml/hr

30. 4.17 ml/min

31. 250 gtt/min

32. 500 min (or 8 hr 20 min)

33. 960 ml

34. 250 min (or 4 hr 10 min)

35. 33 hr 20 min
36. 1 mg/250 ml
37. 4 mcg/ml
38. 40 mcg
39. 80 mg/ml
40. 100 mg or 1.25 ml
41. 120 ml/hr
42. 1 g/500 ml
43. 500 mg/250 ml
44. 50 gtt/min
45. 16 or 17 gtt/min
46. 60 gtt/min
47. 20 gtt/min
48. 62 gtt/min
49. 20 gtt/min
50. 30 gtt/min

CHAPTER 9

1. 4.5 %
2. 3%
3. 36%
4. 27%
5. 13.5%
6. 11%
7. 800 ml/hr (or 6 L 400 ml total)
8. 400 ml (the 12th hour is just one hour)
9. 8.8 mg
10. 3.3 mg
11. 3.25 mg
12. 98.6
13. 38.3
14. −17.8
15. 113
16. 89.6
17. 7.5 ml
18. 3.75 ml
19. 20 ml
20. 5 ml
21. 0.3 ml
22. 10 ml
23. 0.5 m^2
24. 7.61
25. 7.36

CHAPTER 10

Exhibit 10-9: Respiratory Analysis Exercise

alkalosis	−15 Torr
alkalosis	−10 Torr
acidosis	+5 Torr
acidosis	−15 Torr

Exhibit 10-11: Respiratory pH Analysis Exercise

alkalosis	−15 Torr	+0.12 pH
alkalosis	−10 Torr	+0.8 pH
acidosis	+5 Torr	−0.04 pH
acidosis	−15 Torr	−0.12 pH

Exhibit 10-13: pH Change Exercise

alkalosis	0
alkalosis	+0.1
acidosis	−0.08
acidosis	−0.15
alkalosis	+0.15
acidosis	−0.02

Exhibit 10-14: Acid-Base Balance Exercise

0 Torr	0 pH	−.08 pH	−0.08 pH
0 Torr	0 pH	−0.15 pH	−0.15 pH
0 Torr	0 pH	−0.25 pH	−0.25 pH
0 Torr	0 pH	−0.20 pH	−0.20 pH
10 Torr	−0.08 pH	−0.10 pH	−0.02 pH
10 Torr	−0.08 pH	−0.08 pH	0 pH
10 Torr	−0.08 pH	−0.15 pH	−0.07 pH
10 Torr	−0.08 pH	−0.25 pH	−0.17 pH
10 Torr	−0.08 pH	−0.20 pH	−0.12 pH
10 Torr	−0.08 pH	0 pH	+0.08 pH
-10 Torr	+0.08 pH	0 pH	−0.08 pH
-10 Torr	+0.08 pH	−0.10 pH	−0.18 pH
-10 Torr	+0.08 pH	−0.08 pH	−0.16 pH
-10 Torr	+0.08 pH	−0.15 pH	−0.23 pH
-10 Torr	+0.08 pH	−0.25 pH	−0.33 pH
-10 Torr	+0.08 pH	−0.20 pH	−0.28 pH

Review Problems

1. −0.10 pH
2. 0 pH
3. −0.10 pH
4. 15 mEq/L
5. 187.5 mEq
6. −0.18 pH
7. −0.08 pH
8. −0.08 pH
9. 5.3 mEq/L
10. 67 mEq
11. −0.10 pH
12. +0.08 pH
13. −0.18 pH
14. 12 mEq/L
15. 150 mEq
16. −0.23 pH
17. 0 pH
18. −0.23 pH
19. 15.3 mEq/L
20. 191 mEq

21. −0.26 pH
22. −0.16 pH
23. −0.10 pH
24. 6.7 mEq/L
25. 141 mEq
26. −0.09 pH
27. −0.04 pH
28. −0.05 pH
29. 4.2 mEq/L
30. 63 mEq
31. +0.04 pH
32. +0.04 pH
33. 0 pH
34 0 mEq/L
35. 0 mEq
36. −0.30 pH
37. 0 pH
38. −0.30 pH
39. 20 mEq/L
40. 375 mEq
41. 0 pH
42. −0.24 pH
43. +0.24 pH
44. 0 mEq/L
45. 0 mEq
46. 0 pH
47. −0.24 pH
48. +0.24 pH
49. −16 mEq/L
50. 0 mEq

Measures, Weights, and Prefixes

HOUSEHOLD MEASURES AND WEIGHTS

1 teaspoon (t)	60 drops (gtt)
	5 milliliters (ml)
	$\frac{1}{8}$ ounce (oz)
	60 minims
	60 grains (gr)
1 tablespoon (T)	3 teaspoons
	$\frac{1}{2}$ fluid ounce
	4 drams
1 cup	16 (fluid) tablespoons
	12 (dry) tablespoons
	8 fluid ounces
1 pint	2 cups
	2 glasses
	16 ounces
	$\frac{1}{2}$ quart

Note: Household units of measure are not precise.

METRIC PREFIXES

Prefix	Unit	Factor
kilo	1,000	one thousand
hecto	100	one hundred
deca	10	ten
deci	0.1	one tenth
centi	$0.01\ (10^{-2})$	one hundredth
milli	$0.000001\ (10^{-6})$	$0.000001\ (10^{-6})$
micro	$0.000001\ (10^{-6})$	one millionth
nano	10^{-9}	one trillionth
pico	10^{-9}	
femto	10^{-9}	
atto	10^{-18}	

Symbols and Abbreviations

SYMBOLS

↑	increased (*not* upper)	=	equal to
↓	decreased (*not* lower)	<	less than
≈	approximately equal to	>	greater than
♂	male	@	at
♀	female	▲	delta symbol meaning "change in/of"

ABBREVIATIONS

A

abd	abdomen
ABG	arterial blood gases
AC	antecubital
A-fib	atrial fibrillation
AIDS	acquired immuno-deficiency syndrome
ALS	advanced life support
AMA	against medical advice
AMI	acute myocardial infarction
APGAR	appearance, pulse, grimace, activity, and respirations scale
approx.	approximately
ASA	acetylsalicylic acid (aspirin)
ASHD	arteriosclerotic heart disease
AV	atrioventricular node

B

BCP	birth control pills
B/F	black female
bicarb	sodium bicarbonate
BID	twice a day
BLS	basic life support
BM	bowel movement
B/M	black male
BOW	bag of waters (amniotic fluid)
BP	blood pressure
BVM	bag valve mask device

C

C	with
°C	degrees Celsius (centigrade)
CA (ca)	cancer
CAD	coronary artery disease
cap	capsule
capt	captain
CBC	complete blood count
cc	cubic centimeter
C/C	chief complaint
C-collar	cervical collar
CCU	coronary care unit
CHF	congestive heart failure
CID	cervical immobilization device
cm	centimeter
CNS	central nervous system
C/O	complained of
CO_2	carbon dioxide
COPD	chronic obstructive pulmonary disease
CPR	cardiopulmonary resuscitation
C-sect	Caesarean section
CSF	cerebrospinal fluid
CV	cardiovascular
CVA	cerebrovascular accident (stroke)

D

D5W	dextrose 5% in water; a solution in which each 100 mL provides 5 gm of Dextrose (number = percent of dextrose)
D50W	50% dextrose in water
D&C	dilatation and curettage
D/C	discontinue
defib	defibrillation

DOA	dead on arrival
DTs	delirium tremens
DX	diagnosis

E

ED	emergency department
EDC	estimated date of confinement (pregnancy due date)
EEG	electroencephalogram
EENT	eyes, ears, nose, and throat
EGTA	esophageal gastric tube airway
EKG	electrocardiogram (ECG)
EMS	emergency medical services
EMT	emergency medical technician
EMT-P	paramedic
ENT	ears, nose, and throat
EOA	esophageal obturator airway
epi	epinephrine
ER	emergency room
ET	endotracheal tube
ETA	estimated time of arrival
ETOH	ethyl alcohol

F

°F	degrees Fahrenheit
fib	fibrillation
fl	fluid
flu	influenza
FUO	fever of unknown origin
Fx	fracture

G

GCS	Glasgow Coma Scale
GI	gastrointestinal

GSW	gunshot wound
gtt	drops

H

Hg	mercury
HIV	human immunodeficiency virus
HL	heparin lock
HPI	history of the present illness (injury)

I

ICS	intercostal space
IM	intramuscular injection
IO	intraosseous infusion
IUD	intrauterine device
IV	intravenous
IVP	intravenous push

J

JVD	jugular vein distention

K

K	potassium
kg	kilogram
KVO	keep vein open (25–30 ml/hr)

L

L	liter
Ⓛ	left
lac	laceration
LBBB	left bundle branch block
L&D	labor and delivery
$L_1 L_2$	lumbar vertebra; numbered 1 through 5 to

	represent their position in the spinal column from proximal to distal in the body
LLQ	left lower quadrant
L/M	liters per minute
LMP	last menstrual period
LOC	level of consciousness
LUQ	left upper quadrant
LVF	left ventricular failure

M

m	meter
MAL	midaxillary line
mcg	microgram (*note:* µg is generally not acceptable unless typed)
MCL	midclavicular line
MD	medical doctor
med	medication
mEq	milliequivalent
mg	milligram
MI	myocardial infarction
min	minute
ml	milliliter
mm	millimeter
MS	morphine sulphate
MSL	midsternal line
MVA	motor vehicle accident
MVC	motor vehicle crash

N

Na	sodium
NaCl	sodium chloride
NC	nasal cannula
neg	negative
ng	nanogram
NKA	no known allergy
NKDA	no known drug allergy

NPO	nothing per os (by mouth)	PM	afternoon (post-meridiem)
NRB	non-rebreathing oxygen device	PMH	past medical history
NS	normal saline (0.9% sodium chloride solution)	PMI	point of maximal impulse (of the heart)
NSR	normal sinus rhythm	PND	paroxysmal nocturnal dyspnea
NTG	nitroglycerine	PO	per os (by mouth)
N/V	nausea and vomiting	poss.	possible
N/V/D	nausea, vomiting, and diarrhea	POV	privately owned vehicle
		preg.	pregnant
		PRN	as necessary

O

O$_2$	oxygen	Pt.	patient
OB	obstetrical	PTA	prior to arrival
OD	overdose	PVC	premature ventricular contraction
OR	operating room		
oz	ounce		

P

Q

PAC	premature atrial contraction	q	every
		q#h	every # (number of) hours
PARRLA	pupils anisocoric, round, reactive to light, and accommodating	QA	quality assurance
		qd	every day
		qh	every hour
PASG	pneumatic antishock garment	QID	four times a day
PAT	paroxysmal atrial tachy-cardia		

R

PCN	penicillin	Ⓡ	right
PD	police department	RBBB	right bundle branch block
PDR	*Physician's Desk Reference*		
PEA	pulseless electrical activity	RBC	red blood cell
per	by, through	RLQ	right lower quadrant
PERRLA	pupils equal, round, reactive to light, and accommodating	RN	registered nurse
		R/O	rule out
		ROM	range of motion
PID	pelvic inflammatory disease	ROS	review of systems
		rpt	report
PJC	premature junctional contraction	RSR	regular sinus rhythm
		RUQ	right upper quadrant
		Rx	prescription

S

$\overline{S}$	without
SA	sinoatrial node
SIDS	sudden infant death syndrome
SL	sublingually
SNT	soft and not tender
SO	sheriff's office
SOB	shortness of breath
soln	solution
SQ (SC)	subcutaneous injection
stat	at once, instantly
SVT	supraventricular tachycardia

T

tab	tablet
TB	tuberculosis
TIA	transient ischemic attack
TID	three times a day

U

UT	unit (of medication)
URI	upper respiratory tract infection
UTI	urinary tract infection

V

V-fib	ventricular fibrillation
VD	venereal disease
vent	venturi mask
VS	vital signs

W

WBC	white blood cell
W/C	wheelchair
W/D	warm and dry
W/F	white female
W/M	white male
WPW	Wolff-Parkinson White syndrome
W/S	watt seconds (Joules)

X

X	times (as in "repeated four times," not clock times)

Y

Y/O	years old

Glossary

> Philosophy is written in this grand book—I mean the universe—which stands continually open to our gaze, but it cannot be understood unless one first learns to comprehend the language and interpret the characters in which it is written. It is written in the language of mathematics, and its characters are triangles, circles, and other geometrical figures, without which it is humanly impossible to understand a single word of it; without these, one is wandering in a dark labyrinth.
>
> —Galileo, *Il Saggiatore.*

A

absolute value: The positive value of a number regardless of any arithmetic sign attached to it. For example, the absolute value of -6 is $+6$. The absolute value of $+6$ is also $+6$. The absolute value of a number is symbolized by vertical lines placed on either side of the number, as in $|-6|$.

accuracy: The state of being free from mistakes; correctness.

acidosis: A condition in which the blood has a deficit of bicarbonates (base).

acquired tolerance: The development of an increased ability, with repeated exposures, to endure medication; a state where a patient requires more medication, after repeated exposures, to achieve the desired effect.

addiction: The condition of being physically dependent on a substance and having withdrawal symptoms upon cessation of use of the addicting substance.

affect: To act on; to produce an effect or change on something.

alkalosis: A condition in which the bicarbonate (base) levels of the body are higher than normal.

allergy: An unusual sensitivity to a substance. It may be characterized by itching, a rash, wheals, diarrhea, or other systemic reactions.

ampule: A small sealed glass container with a breakable top. It commonly holds one dose of medication.

anaphylactic reaction: An unusual or exaggerated reaction of an individual to a substance; individuals become more susceptible to anaphylaxis with repeated exposures, especially of injected allergens. The reaction results from the internal release of histamines, serotonin, and chemicals. It is also called an "allergic" or "hypersensitive" reaction.

antagonism: Medications that work against each other's effects.

anti: A combining form (prefix) signifying counteraction to the stem word.

antibiotic: An agent that destroys or stops the growth of bacteria.

antidepressant: A classification of medication that is used to treat psychological depression, usually by depressing the central nervous system.

antidote: A remedy for counteracting a poison or the toxic effects of a medication.

antidysrhythmic: An agent or treatment that acts to suppress cardiac dysrhythmia.

antihistamine: An agent that is used to minimize the effect of histamine in allergic conditions.

antihyperglycemic: An agent that counteracts high levels of glucose in the blood.

antihypertensive: A classification of medication that is used to treat abnormally high blood pressure.

antihypoglycemic: A classification of medication that is used to stimulate secretion of insulin in diabetic patients. It is usually an orally administered medication.

apothecary system: A system of measurement that originated in England.

Arabic number system: The counting system commonly used throughout the modern world; it uses the base 10 and numeric characters of 0, 1, 2, 3, 4, 5, 6, 7, 8, and 9.

B

balance: To have multiple parts in equilibrium.

barbiturate: A sedative medication derived from a barbiturate acid. Barbiturates are considered highly addictive.

base: Mathematically, a constant figure on which mathematical values are computed, as in logarithms; in logarithms, where the logarithm is the exponent and the base is the number that is to be raised to the value of the exponent; physiologically, a compound that will react with an acid to form a salt or a compound that will dissolve in solution to form hydroxyl (OH^-) ions.

behavioral toxicity: A person who is under the influence of a medication and may take actions that could cause harm or death to the person. An example is a person who jumps from a fatal height believing he can fly.

body temperature: A measurement of the temperature of the human body. Normal body temperature is 98.6°F, or 37°C.

boiling point: A measurement of the temperature at which a liquid will boil and convert to a gas. Boiling point of water is 212°F, or 100°C.

bolus: A lump or mass of something that is all in one part. An intravenous bolus is the administration of fluid medication all in one injection, as opposed to mixing with and dripping through another IV solution.

C

carbonic acid: The acid created by dissolving carbon dioxide in solution under pressure. It is a weak acid that easily breaks down to carbon dioxide and water when the pressure is removed.

cardiotonic: An agent that affects cardiac contractility or rate.

Celsius: A designation of the metric temperature scale, named after Swedish astronomer Anders Celsius, on which 0° is the freezing point of water and 100° is the boiling point of water under laboratory conditions.

centi: A combining form (prefix) indicating a metric division by 100 of the combined unit, as in *centimeter*, which is one hundredth of a meter.

centigrade: Referring to the Celsius temperature scale. It was the preferred term until the adoption of *Celsius* by an international conference on weights and measures in 1948.

chemical name: A name for a chemical that is based on its physical structure. For example, water's chemical name is dihydrogen oxide.

chemotherapy: The treatment of illness or disease by administration of chemicals.

chronotropic: An agent that affects the cardiac rate.

colloid: A fluid in which substances (such as proteins) are mixed; not a true solution; it generally will not diffuse through a semipermeable membrane.

compensate: In medicine, to counterbalance a defect in the function of a part or system by increased activity by another part or system.

concentration: The strength or density, as in a solution.

concomitant: Occurring at the same time; taking two medications at the same time.

confidentiality: Patients have a right to privacy regarding their medical records.

correct: To set right; when a physiological deficit in a body system returns to normal action (as opposed to *compensate*).

cross multiply: A two-step method of solving ratio equations by first multiplying both sides of the equation by the product of the denominators of both sides and then by dividing both sides by the coefficient of the unknown.

crystalloid: A substance that dissolves in solution and can then diffuse through a semipermeable membrane.

cubic centimeter: A metric measurement that is equivalent in volume to 1 ml.

D

deci: A combining form (prefix) indicating a metric measurement that is divided by 10, as in decimeter (one tenth of a meter).

decimal: A fraction or mixed number with the fraction expressed with a denominator that is a power of 10. The numerator is written and the denominator is omitted but indicated as a factor of 10 with a point placed to the left of the numerator to indicate the denominator's value. For example, 7/100 is 0.07.

deka: A combining form (prefix) indicating a metric measurement that is multiplied by 10, as in decameter (10 meters).

denominator: The number placed below (or to the right of) the line in fractions that shows into how many equal parts the whole is divided.

dependence: The psychological and/or physical state of addiction in which the user must continue or increase usual doses of a drug to prevent withdrawal symptoms.

depot: The physical location in the body in which a drug or medication is stored.

depressant: An agent that diminishes function; generically, a central nervous system depressant, but a cardiac depressant diminishes cardiac function, etc.

dilution: A substance that has been made less concentrated.

dimension: An extension in a single line or direction as length, breadth, and height or extent, size, and degree. In physics, a fundamental quantity, such as mass, length, or time, is measured like all other physical quantities, such as those of area, velocity, and power.

dimensional analysis: To perform calculations to compare one dimension to another. In dosage calculations, one can compare and contrast diverse units of measure to identify doses to be titrated, rapidly IV bolused, slowly infused, slowly bolused, injected, given by mouth, inhaled, adsorbed through the skin, or given by suppository.

diuretic: A medication that increases urinary discharge.

division: To separate into pieces.

dividend: That which is to be divided; in a fraction, the numerator (the number on top).

divisor: The number by which the dividend is being divided to produce the quotient.

dose: The quantity of medication given at one time.

dose related effect: The effects that change rather than increase with increasing dosages of a medication.

E

effect: That which is produced by a cause; the result of a dose of medication.

elixir: A medicine consisting of a sweetened alcoholic solution of a drug.

endotracheal instillation: A route of the administration of medication in which medication is instilled directly into the endotracheal tube of a patient.

equation: An expression made up of two parts connected by an equal sign (=).

ethics: The study of right and wrong.

exponent: A number written above the line of the rest of the text (superscripted), indicating how many times the base is multiplied by itself. The exponent of 10^2 is 2, the exponent of 10^3 is 3, etc.

extracellular fluid: Fluid that is found outside cells; it accounts for one third of total body water and includes intravascular and interstitial fluids.

F

factor (noun): One of the two or more parts that, when multiplied together, form a given product, as in "2" and "3" and "mg," which are all factors of "6 mg."

factor (verb): To resolve an expression into its factors.

Fahrenheit: A unit of temperature measure, named after the German physicist Gabriel Daniel Fahrenheit (1686–1736). The Fahrenheit scale registers 32° as the freezing point of water, 98.6° as normal human body temperature, and 212° as the boiling point of water.

FDA: The federal Food and Drug Administration, a division of the U.S. Department of Health and Human Services. The FDA is responsible for approving new medications and foods offered for sale in the United States.

first pass effect: A phenomenon in which an orally administered medication normally enters the digestive portal circulation system, is routed through the liver, and is metabolized by the normal function of the liver, significantly reducing its pharmacokinetic potency.

flow rate: The rate of administration of an intravenous solution, calculated in drops per minute or milliliters per hour.

formula: A set of mathematic symbols expressing a fact—for example, area = 2π radius^2 is the formula for the area of a circle; a description of the composition of a chemical (medication).

fraction: A mathematical expression signifying division; two numbers are divided by a horizontal line or by a vertical slanted line. The number above (or to the left of) the line is the numerator. The part below the line is the denominator.

freezing point: The temperature at which water freezes, which is 32 degrees Fahrenheit and 0 degrees Celsius.

G

g: The metric abbreviation for *gram*.

generic name: The name given under standard naming conventions that reflects the medication's molecular structure. All chemicals have several names (*see also* chemical name and trade name).

golden rules: The rules of acid base balance are based on the Henderson–Hasselbalch equation and are unit conversion factors between pH, Torr, and milliequivalents of extra-cellular body fluid.

gr: The abbreviation for *grain*, a household unit of measure.

gram: The metric unit of mass. It is equivalent to 15.432 gr, or 0.035 oz avoirdupois. It is abbreviated *g*.

H

habituation: The gradual adaptation to repeated doses of medication. There may be psychological dependence but no true addiction to the medication.

half-life: The time in which a medication is metabolized by the body and becomes one half as pharmaceutically active as when administered.

hallucinogen: An agent that causes the patient to have false perceptions. The perceptions can be visual, auditory, or felt.

hecto: A combining form (prefix) indicating a multiplication by 100 of the combined unit. A hectogram is 100 g.

hypersensitivity: A state of having an exaggerated response to a medication.

hypertonic: Having a greater osmotic pressure than body fluid (0.9% solute).

hypnotic: A medication that induces sleep.

hypotonic: Having a lesser osmotic pressure than body fluid; a solution that will enter the body cells and may cause hemolysis (the breakdown of red blood cells).

I

improper fraction: A fraction in which the numerator is larger than the denominator; a fraction that is not reduced to its lowest terms.

informed consent: Given by the patient after he knows all the possible risks.

infusion: An introduction of a medication into the body, usually by intravenous therapy.

inotropic: An agent that has a effect on cardiac contraction. If it causes stronger contractions, it is considered a positive inotropic effect. If it causes weaker concentrations, it has a negative inotropic effect.

inscription: The body of the prescription.

integer: A whole number.

intracardiac: Relating to an injection into the inside of the heart.

intracellular fluid: Water within the cells of the body; accounts for two thirds of the total body water.

intradermal: Identifies a location between the layers of skin. Some injections are given subcutaneously into the intradermal layers.

intramuscular: Relating to an injection into the inside of a muscle.

intraosseous: An intraosseous (IO) injection is injected directly into the bone. A child's leg and an adult's sternum are the most popular sites for IO injections.

intravenous: Relating to an injection or infusion into the inside of a vein.

invert: To turn upside down.

isotonic: Refers to a solution that has the same concentration of electrolytes as blood. There is no strong osmosis or diffusion between an isotonic solution and blood.

K

kilo: A combining form (prefix) indicating a multiplication by 1,000 of the combined unit; a kilogram is 1,000 g.

kilogram: A metric unit of mass equivalent to the weight of 1 deciliter (1,000 cc) of sterile, fluid water at sea level, 0°C (32°F), and standard atmospheric pressure; equal to 2.204623 lb.

KVO: An intravenous infusion rate calculated to be fast enough to prevent blood clotting on the catheter; approximately 25 to 30 ml per hour.

L

liter: A metric unit of volume equal to 1,000 cc.

log: An abbreviation for *logarithm*.

logarithm: The exponent of the power to which a fixed number, the base, is raised to produce the number, the antilogarithm. The common logarithm system uses a base of 10.

lowest common denominator: The simplest denominator held in common among a group of fractions. Fractions must be scaled to larger or smaller fractions with a commonly held denominator for addition or subtraction. The lowest common denominator that can be used to add $1/4$ and $1/3$ is 12. So $1/4$ would be scaled up to $3/12$, and $1/3$ would be scaled up to $4/12$. The sum of those two fractions is $7/12$.

M

mass: The characteristic of a body that gives it inertia. For the purpose of dosage calculations, it may be considered weight; however, this is a simplification of the scientific definition of mass.

mcg: The standard metric abbreviation for *microgram*.

MedicAlert: A trade name for a bracelet or necklace that bears medical information about the wearer.

medicine: Any drug or remedy; any medicine may be toxic when taken in incorrect doses.

mega: A combining form (prefix) indicating 1,000,000 of the combined unit.

mEq: Abbreviation for *milliequivalents*; the standard metric unit of measure for electrolytic (ionic) solutions.

meter: The standard metric unit of measure for length.

metric system: An international system of measurements; also known as the International System of Units.

mg: The standard metric abbreviation for *milligram*, one thousandth of a gram.

micro: A combining form (prefix) indicating small size; one millionth (10^{-6}) of the combined unit.

milli: A combining form (prefix) indicating a metric unit of measure of one thousandth (10^{-3}) of the combined unit.

milliequivalent: The concentration of electrolytes in solution, usually measured in milliequivalent per liter.

mineral origin: Made from vitamins and minerals.

mixed number: A number expressed as a whole number and a fraction.

mixture: A combination of two or more substances without a chemical bond causing them to combine to form a new molecule.

mixture rule: The titration is always equal to the sum of the medication and the water.

mucosa: Include the tongue, gums, cheeks, vaginal walls, and, in general, body parts that remain wet and may be a route of infection for a contagious disease to enter the body.

multiplication: The process of finding a product (answer) by repeating a specified quantity (multiplicand) a specified number of times (multiplier); indicated in mathematics by an *x* or asterisk "*" or parenthesis marks "( )" or brackets "[ ]" or braces "{ }"; when several sets of multiplication are to be performed in one expression, the order of operations is to work from the innermost set of multipliers to the outermost.

N

nano: A combining form (prefix) indicating a metric measurement of one billionth (10^{-9}) of the combined unit.

narcotic: A habit-forming medication that depresses the central nervous system and induces sleep and anesthesia. Excessive doses produce coma and death. Examples include heroin, morphine, codeine, and many synthetics.

negative log: A logarithm that represents a fraction of the number 1 divided by the logarithm; the inverse of a positive logarithm.

negative: A quantity less than zero.

nonparenteral: A medication that is administered through the alimentary canal—that is, taken orally or by rectal suppository.

numerator: In a fraction, the number on top; the dividend; the number to be divided.

O

order of operations: The sequence in which mathematical operations are done when more than one mathematical step is required for solution of a problem. When markers such as braces, brackets, or parentheses are used, the operation inside the markers is performed first. When division or multiplication are indicated, order of operations between these two operations does not matter. When division or multiplication is indicated with addition or subtraction in the same problem, the multiplication and/or division is performed first.

organic: Relating to matter that is or was at one time a living organism.

overdose: A dose of a drug that is sufficient to cause an acute reaction such as coma, mania, hysteria, or death; too large of a dose.

P

Pa: In the measurement of arterial blood gases, Pa refers to the partial pressure of a gas in arterial blood (i.e., pressure arterial).

parenteral: Indicating any route other than the alimentary canal, such as intravenous, intra-arterial, intracardiac, mucosal, inhalation, adsorption, etc.

patient weight: The weight of the person receiving medicinal care; the *ideal* weight of the person receiving medicinal care.

PDR: Abbreviation for *Physician's Desk Reference*, an *unofficial* reference text for medications sold in the United States.

percent: A number with a percent sign (%) indicating a quantity per 100. For example, 20 per 100 (20/100) is 20%.

percutaneous: Penetrating through the skin.

pH: The potential of hydrogen; the symbol for the negative logarithm (inverse logarithm) indicating hydrogen ion concentration in solution. pH indicates the acidity or alkalinity of a solution: 7.0 is neutral; 7.36 to 7.44 is normal for the human body. pH values of 6.9 (on the acidic side) and 7.8 (on the alkaline side) are incompatible with human life.

plunger: The shaft of a syringe that, when pushed, expels the medication.

positive: An integer; a quantity greater than zero.

potentiation: The synergistic action of two or more substances in which the total effects are greater than the sum of the independent effects of the two substances.

precision: The quality of being precise or minutely exact.

product: The answer in a multiplication problem; see *multiplication*.

proportion: An equality between two or more ratios. For example, 12 is to 1 dozen as 6 is to $1/2$ dozen.

Q

quotient: The number obtained when one quantity is divided by another.

R

rate: A ratio that deals with units of time—that is, units of medication per units of time.

ratio: A constant relationship of one quantity to another. For example, there are 10 mg/ml.

reciprocal: The reciprocal of any quantity is the quotient of 1 divided by the quantity. For example, the reciprocal of 2 is $1/2$.

recombinant DNA therapy: A therapy of modifying DNA (genes) or an organism to produce characteristics not normally found; also known as "gene splicing." Recombinant therapy has been used to stimulate bacteria and yeast to produce medications such as human insulin.

reconstitution: The process of mixing sterile water and a powdered medication, which is stored dry, to generate an injectable solution of a medication.

relative base deficit: In acid-base balance calculations, the amount of base needed to achieve balance; this is independent of the cause of the acid-base imbalance—that is, whether it is too little base or too much acid.

Rule of Nines: A formula by which the amount of body surface affected by a burn may be calculated by assigning major parts of the body values of 9%. The Rule of Nines is not the same for adults and small children.

S

scale: A graduated or proportioned measure, such as the pH scale.

serum: A medication prepared from blood products of humans or animals; the watery portion of the blood.

side effect: An action or effect of a medication other than the primary one for which it was administered. A side effect may be untoward (undesired) or desired.

For example, some antihistamines have a side effect of drowsiness. If you take one at bedtime intending to sleep, this becomes a desired side effect. The same side effect in different circumstances, such as driving your car to work, would become an untoward effect because it may cause a driver to fall asleep at the wheel.

sign: An observable, objective, measurable, finite evidence about a patient (as opposed to symptoms, which the patient reports to the clinician).

signature: Includes the physician's signature and instructions for the patient as well as other general information.

solute: A substance that is dissolved in solution.

solution: A liquid containing a dissolved substance (solute).

solvent: The liquid into which a substance is placed to create a solution; water is considered the universal solvent.

stimulant: Generally increases the effects of whatever organ or system to which it is administered.

subcutaneous: Beneath the skin; referring to a route of administration of medication by injection. Subcutaneous injection has the slowest rate of adsorption of all routes of injection.

sublingual: Underneath the tongue; referring to a route of administration of medication for adsorption by mucosal membranes.

subscription: Directions to the pharmacist about preparing the medication.

sum: The result obtained by adding two or more numbers.

superscription: The Rx symbol.

suppository: A semisolid substance to be placed into the rectum, vagina, or urethra, where it dissolves.

symbol: A sign that represents a quantity or unit of measure by association.

synergism: The harmonious action of two medications producing an effect greater than the sum of the independent effects of the medications.

synthetic origin: Manufactured in a laboratory.

syringe: A tubular device that, when attached to a needle, may be used to contain and administer medication by injection.

syrup: A medication in a concentrated solution of sugar and water used primarily to give medications pleasant taste and odor.

T

therapeutic: Having a healing effect.

therapeutic envelope: A range from a minimum dose to a maximum dose within which a medication has a beneficial effect. Below the therapeutic envelope, the dose is "subtherapeutic" and will have no beneficial effect. Above the therapeutic envelope, the dose may have toxic effects and cause "overdose."

threshold: A point at which effects begin to be produced.

titration: The concentration of a chemical solution; a concentration that produces a desired effect.

tolerance: The capacity to endure medication without adverse effect; sensitivity to medication.

Torr: A metric unit of measure for a substance that exerts the pressure sufficient to elevate a column of mercury in a vertical tube 1 ml high under standard atmospheric pressure. The Torr is used to measure gases that exert pressure.

total body surface area: A calculation of the square area of the skin of the body.

toxic: Poisonous; interfering with normal physiological function.

trade name: The name a pharmaceutical company gives its medication to enhance marketability. For example, many Americans refer to facial tissue (generic name) as Kleenex (trade name) because Kleenex has become synonymous with facial tissue.

tranquilizers: Agents that have a depressant effect on the central nervous system.

U

unit conversion factor: A ratio proportion between two different units of measure; it is equal to the whole number 1. For example, "12 to 1 dozen" may be expressed as a fraction (12/1 dozen) or proportion (12:1 dozen).

unit of measure: A determined amount adopted as a standard of measurement.

unknown: A quantity in a mathematical expression that is not known and is represented by a symbol.

untoward effect: A generic description of effects that are not therapeutic in a given individual; these include (but are not necessarily) hypersensitive, allergic, or unexpected effects. For example, a side effect of antihistamines (often taken for colds) is drowsiness. If a patient is in bed, trying to rest, that side effect is therapeutic. However, if the patient is trying to work or drive an automobile, that side effect is not good and is "untoward."

V

vaccine: A medication given to patients who have not yet contracted a disease. It is intended to generate illness-specific antibodies before the patient is exposed so when and if a patient is exposed to the disease, his immune system can defeat the disease.

variable: The unknown factor in an equation.

vasopressor: An agent that acts to affect an increase in blood pressure. They act several different ways.

vial: A small glass container with a rubber stopper in the top that contains multiple doses of a medication.

volume: The space occupied by a substance.

W

water soluble: A substance that will dissolve in water (and blood serum).

whole number: An integer as opposed to a fraction or mixed number.

withdrawal: Symptoms associated with abstention from a drug to which an individual has become physically addicted.

word factor: A factor that is not an integer (*see also* factor).

Index